# The *Diabetic Woman*

# The Diabetic Woman

Lois Jovanovic-Peterson, M.D.

June Biermann

Barbara Toohey

*A Jeremy P. Tarcher/Putnam Book*

Published by G. P. Putnam's Sons
New York

Most Tarcher/Putnam books are available at special quantity discounts for bulk purchases for sales promotions, premiums, fund-raising, and educational needs. Special books or book excerpts also can be created to fit specific needs.

For details, write or telephone Special Markets, The Putnam Publishing Group, 200 Madison Avenue, New York, NY 10016; (212) 951-8891.

"The Night Mom Lost It at Friendly's" by Nancy Aronie; used by permission.

Exercise illustrations from *Diabetes: Your Complete Exercise Guide* (pp. 29–31) by Neil F. Gordon, Champaign, IL: Human Kinetics Publishers. Copyright 1993 by Neil F. Gordon. Reprinted by permission.

"Ten Commandments for Avoiding Negative Scenes with Diabetic Loved Ones" reprinted with permission from *Psyching Out Diabetes* by Richard R. Rubin, Ph.D., June Biermann and Barbara Toohey, © 1993, RGA Publishing Group, Inc.

Illustration of MiniMed Pump courtesy of Grey Zone Creative Services.

Illustration of Autopen courtesy of Owen Mumford, Inc.

Illustration of Novolin Pen © 1995 Novo Nordisk Pharmaceuticals, Inc.

A Jeremy P. Tarcher/Putnam Book
Published by G. P. Putnam's Sons
*Publishers Since 1838*
200 Madison Avenue
New York, NY 10016
http://www.putnam.com/putnam

LIBRARY OF CONGRESS CATALOGING-IN-PUBLICATION DATA

Jovanovic-Peterson, Lois.
    The diabetic woman / Lois Jovanovic-Peterson, June Biermann, Barbara Toohey.
        p.   cm.
    "A Jeremy P. Tarcher/Putnam book"
    Includes index.
    ISBN 0-87477-829-8
    1. Diabetes—Popular works.  2. Women—Diseases.  3. Diabetes in pregnancy—Popular works.  I. Biermann, June.  II. Toohey, Barbara.
III. Title.
RC660.4.J675   1996              616.4′62′0082—dc20              95-49952   CIP

Book design by Patrice Sheridan
Cover design by Mauna Eichner

Printed in the United States of America

    3   4   5   6   7   8   9   10

This book is printed on acid-free paper. ∞

To my dear husband, Dr. Charles M. Peterson,
who loves me despite and because of my
(and his) diabetes.
Thank you for motivating me to take care of
myself. And to Kevin and Larisa and Boyce for
sharing it all with me.

—L. J.-P.

# Contents

# _Preface to the Second Edition

IN THE NINE YEARS SINCE THE PUBLICATION OF THE FIRST edition of *The Diabetic Woman*, we've received numerous letters from women expressing their gratitude that a book addressing their unique problems had been written and telling the positive impact on their lives of what they learned from it. After first asking "Where can I find a doctor in my area who is exactly like Dr. Lois?" (sorry, she's one of a kind), virtually every letter contained a plea for more—more answers to their specific questions, coverage of more subjects, more details on the subjects that were covered. We always responded to their letters, asking Dr. Lois for answers to the questions that only a doctor of her life and professional experience could answer. Sometimes we published Dr. Lois's responses in *The Diabetic Reader*, but as our file of questions grew, we realized all the answers should be made available to the women who needed them.

One area in which the questioning was heaviest was

that of pregnancy. Although we had discussed the subject in the first edition, women were thirsting for more information. We had given them a sip; they wanted a whole bucketful. As good fortune would have it, pregnancy is one of Dr. Lois's prime areas of interest and expertise; and in the last eight years she has developed into a national leader in that field, even, in 1995, winning the prestigious American Diabetes Association's Outstanding Clinician in Diabetes Award for her achievements. We've prevailed upon her to add to this edition two whole supplements: one on Type I pregnancies and one on gestational diabetes.

Along with providing answers to more questions, we knew it was time to update a lot of the information in the first edition. The Diabetes Control and Complication Trial has proven that good control does prevent complications, and new products and techniques have been developed to make that control easier to achieve. New dietary guidelines are starting to relax the formerly rigid—and stringent—rules of the past. It's all good news, and we wanted to deliver it so diabetic women everywhere could enjoy and benefit from the positive changes.

But one thing hasn't changed: the basic message of the original book. It's odd, but we didn't even know what the message was. A couple of years ago, a woman was telling June how much the book had meant to her and how it had influenced her. June asked her what was the most important thing she'd learned from the book. . . . Was it how to handle her pregnancy? The influence of hormones on blood sugar? Techniques for achieving good control? The woman thought a moment and said, "All that was valuable, of course, but the most important thing the book taught me was that I have to be a little more selfish."

That message is one thing we haven't changed.

June Biermann
Barbara Toohey
Van Nuys, California
1995

# The Diabetic Woman

# $\mathscr{C}$herchez la Femme

## *June Biermann and Barbara Toohey*

BECAUSE WE'VE WRITTEN EIGHT BOOKS ON DIABETES, PEO-
ple often write to us suggesting other books that are
needed and that they wish we would write. The one
book that has been suggested over and over is a book on
the woman diabetic, on how to handle all the unique
problems of being a diabetic along with all the unique
problems of being a woman.

We realized the need but frankly didn't feel capable of
the task. For all our previous books we used June as the
guinea pig, telling about her diagnosis and coming to
terms with diabetes in *The Peripatetic Diabetic*, answering
all the basic questions about diabetes and diabetes therapy in *The Diabetic's Book*, reporting her experiences and
those of other sports-minded, active diabetics in *The Diabetic's Sports and Exercise Book*, and presenting an approach concentrating on health rather than illness in *The
Diabetic's Total Health Book*.

We felt confident and capable in those areas, but June
just didn't have the total experience necessary for us to

*1*

counsel all women with diabetes. Since her diabetes was diagnosed at age forty-five, she couldn't describe what it was like to go through the upheavals of puberty while trying to keep diabetes in control, nor could she describe what it was like to be a young wife juggling diabetes along with all her other growing responsibilities. June had no children—and if she had, she would have had them before becoming diabetic and thus could not make any personal contributions on that most crucial issue of how a diabetic woman has a successful pregnancy. She couldn't even give firsthand reports about going through menopause, because she'd had a hysterectomy a year before her diabetes was discovered. (We've often thought that the hysterectomy might have been the stress that pulled the trigger on her diabetes-loaded genetic gun.)

No, we definitely didn't have the experiential where-withal needed for a book on the diabetic woman. We often discussed the issue. What we really had to have, we finally decided, was a collaborator. That ideal collabora-tor would be a diabetic woman endocrinologist specializ-ing in diabetes. She would need to be up-to-date on the latest developments in the field, but she shouldn't be so fresh from her residency that she wouldn't have the in-depth background of having worked with a large number of patients. We wanted her to be married, and we wanted her to have children—and to have given birth to them while she was a diabetic. We wanted her to be a warm and compassionate person who would have empa-thy for every problem—no matter how minor it might seem—that a diabetic woman could have. We wanted her to be a clear thinker and a graceful writer with a practical turn of mind. We wanted her to be someone oriented toward working with people, not strictly a re-searcher who looked at everything in terms of studies done with rats. And we wanted her to have a sense of humor—we knew we could never work with someone who didn't have that!

Even we had to laugh at our outrageous demands. How could we ever expect to find such a paragon? Eternal optimists that we are, though, we started broadcasting it around that we were trying to find the name of a diabetic woman diabetologist. We didn't go into all the other requirements we had. Even so, we heard nothing; apparently, not even a shadow of the person we needed existed. We pushed the project to the back of our minds.

Nevertheless, our women readers kept asking questions, so we kept muttering to friends in the diabetes health professions that we sure wished we could find a diabetic woman physician specializing in diabetes. One day our mutterings and our prayers were answered. A Novo Nordisk Insulin representative Tom Avery asked, "Isn't Lois Jovanovic-Peterson a diabetic woman?" and then, answering his own question, he said, "Yes, I'm sure she is."

Our first lead! Although Dr. Jovanovic-Peterson was on the East Coast and we were on the West, her name was familiar to us. We thought we remembered that she worked with the eminent diabetologist Dr. Charles Peterson (now her husband) at Rockefeller University. This was confirmed when we received a copy of their new book, *The Diabetes Self-Care Method*, which doctors Peterson and Jovanovic had written together. We were extremely impressed by the book and excited by the fact that Dr. Jovanovic-Peterson was a good writer and collaborator. Although nowhere in the book was it mentioned that one of the authors actually was a diabetic woman, we were particularly attracted by one illustration, a close-up of four pristine-looking fingertips. The caption was: "These are the tips of the fingers of a diabetic person who for the past eight years has monitored her own blood glucose." We suspected whose fingertips they were.

All these seemed like sufficiently good omens for us to begin our tentative "collaboration mating dances" with Dr. Jovanovic-Peterson. We asked our editor to get in touch and see if she might be interested in working with us, because we didn't want her to feel put on the spot, as she would be if we asked her directly. The answer was that she was not only very enthusiastic about the idea of the collaboration but, according to our editor, she had also said that she had enjoyed our books. That took care of the sense of humor problem. No physician without one would have the slightest taste for our writing.

As we got closer to the collaboration, we received a biographical sketch that revealed her credentials to be even beyond our original outrageous demands: B.S. in Biology from Columbia University; M.D. from Albert Einstein College of Medicine; intern and resident in internal medicine at New York Hospital; research fellow in endocrinology and metabolism at Cornell University Medical College, and later instructor and then associate professor in obstetrics/gynecology at that same institution; guest investigator at Rockefeller University; and soon, as convenience would have it, she was moving west to be senior scientist at the Sansum Medical Research Foundation in Santa Barbara—near us. She'd also written enough professional articles on diabetes to choke a library. We later found out that, in addition to all of the above, as a physician she had been involved with more than 130 diabetic pregnancies (half of which resulted in babies named Lois!). And *two* of the pregnancies she had been involved with were her own. Bingo.

And so it happened that despite the fact that we'd never met Dr. Jovanovic-Peterson face-to-face, we agreed to collaborate on *The Diabetic Woman*. Our first meeting with Lois—as we had come to think of her—took place in New York at the American Diabetes Association's 33rd Postgraduate Course where she was a featured speaker.

When we first saw Lois, we realized that her age was exactly as we had ordered. She was youthful—probably in her early thirties—and, except for the braid, she looked like the description of her written by Gennell Subak-Sharpe in the book *Living With Diabetes:* "Dr. Jovanovic arrives, looking more like a pert schoolgirl than a doctor, with her long dark hair worn in a single braid and a brightly colored scarf tied around her waist." And she was obviously experienced. We were awed by her presentation at the meeting, as well as her responses to questions from the audience—smooth, lucid, and fraught with information. Here was a woman who had it all in her head and right at her fingertips, to mix metaphors.

Although we had confidence at this point that Lois was right for the book, it wasn't until a few weeks later that for us the whipped cream was put on the collaborative sundae.

We had written to ask Lois some specific questions. When she called she apologized for not getting in touch sooner, explaining that she'd had to go to the office to use the phone because her new puppy had chewed through the telephone cord. "What kind of dog do you have?" asked Barbara (with visions frolicking in her head of something appropriately exotic for a noted endocrinologist: a Lhasa apso, maybe, or a komondor).

"Oh, I don't know what she is," Lois replied. "I just went to the pound and took the first puppy who licked my face."

At that moment, we knew for sure that we'd found our woman—and yours.

# $\mathcal{T}$rue Confessions

*Lois Jovanovic-Peterson, M.D.*

MY FATHER HAD TYPE I DIABETES. BY THE TIME HE HAD CHILdren, he was already riddled with problems. I remember his morning ritual of testing his urine—with a tablet, which I now know was Clinitest. The test tube became very hot, and the contents then turned an ugly brown or orange. Now I realize that he never, never was in good control. He took his insulin with a glass syringe, which mother boiled. Every afternoon he had an insulin reaction (insulin shock caused by extremely low blood sugar), and if we didn't rush home from school to give him dinner, he was in a diabetic coma.

From my earliest memories, Daddy was bedridden and blind. At the time of his death, I was twelve; he was fifty, with twenty years of diabetes. I promised at his graveside that I would devote my life to curing diabetes.

At almost the exact age at which my father got his diabetes, I developed mine. I had completed medical school and medical residency and was in the middle of my endocrine/metabolism fellowship when it happened to me.

I completely denied the symptoms. I attributed my weight loss, irritability, and insomnia (which was caused by my constant need to urinate during the night) to the stress of my career.

Then, during the middle of an experiment, I donated my blood as a normal control. When it came back sky-high—more than three times the normal range—I thought the assay was wrong. When my blood was used to calibrate the biostator (a kind of giant mechanical pancreas used in hospitals), I did not think that the 400 blood sugar might be mine but instead screamed at the technician that she was not calibrating the machine correctly.

After three months of deteriorating health, I was forced by a dear friend and colleague to accept the truth. I refused, however, to admit that I needed insulin. I was sure that I could manage my "mild diabetes" with diet (in essence, starvation), exercise, and, if necessary, oral agents. In less than a week I was in a ketoacidotic coma, that advanced state of out-of-control diabetes that can lead to death if insulin is not given.

Denial was certainly the major component in the onset of my diabetes. The next stages were all in accordance with the classic stages described in Elisabeth Kübler-Ross's book *On Death and Dying*. I went through the phases of anger and depression and finally arrived at recovery and acceptance. This process took me a year. Now I know that a year of grief is normal when a chronic disease is diagnosed.

I didn't really change my career plans, but I refused to "come out of the closet." The truth was difficult to admit publicly. I thought my credibility as a physician and a scientist would be harmed. I only revealed my diabetes five years ago, when I went on a big, big insulin pump. Then I *couldn't* deny my "affliction"!

Surprisingly, I found out that my diabetes actually enhanced my credibility. Not only were physicians more respectful but in addition patients became more willing to follow my advice, since they knew I was following it myself.

Perhaps my acceptance took too long—but then again, I saw my father crippled by the disease, and thus it was terrifying to me. And it did serve to make me understanding of denial in other diabetic people and to allow me to be better able to help them work through theirs.

I haven't cured diabetes, nor has anyone else—yet. I have all faith, though, that someone will find a cure in the not-too-distant future. In the meantime, your goal should be to stay healthy and to keep your blood sugar normal so that you'll be ready to enjoy the benefits of that cure. Your other goal should be to lead a wonderful life. What, after all, is the good of being a perfect diabetic woman if it means sacrificing all the joys of human existence?

I know from my own personal experience, as June knows from hers, that these two goals—good control and a wonderful life—are not incompatible. They *can* be achieved. My goal in this book is to help you achieve them.

# 1 ❧ *W*hat Every Diabetic Woman Should Know

WE DON'T THINK OF THIS BOOK AS BEING DIRECTED SPECIFI-
cally to the woman who knows nothing or next to nothing about diabetes. (See Recommended Reading in
Appendix A for a list of good, easy-to-read basic books
for the beginning diabetic woman.) Still, we realize that
some newly diagnosed women are very likely to come
across this book and read it before reading any other.
Therefore, we want to start off with a brief rundown of
the what's, who's, and why's of diabetes. This may also
be good information for women who have had diabetes
for quite a while but who may have some ideas that are
out of date or even flat-out wrong. As the rustic philosopher Josh Billings put it, "It iz better tew know nothing
than tew know what ain't so."

After a brief review of the basics, we'll go on to a
discussion of the questions that concern every woman
with diabetes, no matter what age she may be or what
kind of life she may be leading: active or passive; career

outside the home, inside the home, or both; married, single, or divorced; mother or not.

Dr. Lois, please lead off by telling us just what this thing called diabetes is.

**DR. LOIS:** Diabetes mellitus means "flowing of honey." It refers to the copious amount of urine produced when the blood glucose (level of sugar in the bloodstream) is high. Diabetes mellitus is, therefore, the name given to a disease characterized by a high blood-sugar level.

**JUNE AND BARBARA:** Just how high is high enough for a person to be categorized as diabetic?

**DR. LOIS:** The diagnosis of diabetes is usually based on a glucose-tolerance test. This test consists of 75 grams of sugar given as a drink, with blood tests drawn before the drink and one, two, and three hours after it.

The arbitrary cutoff established by the National Diabetes Data Group in 1979 stated that diabetes mellitus is defined as a fasting plasma glucose above 140 milligrams per deciliter (mg/dl) and/or any plasma glucose that is above 200 mg/dl after two or three hours have elapsed.

With these levels as the cutoffs, anyone whose blood-sugar levels are higher receives the label of "diabetic." How the blood sugars became high is another matter.

If the blood sugar rose because the person's pancreas failed to secrete enough insulin, then the person is classified as a Type I diabetic person. If the person has a high blood-sugar level because she or he cannot get rid of the sugar once it's ingested—in other words, has a clearance problem—then the person has Type II diabetes.

Two other forms of diabetes are possible. Gestational diabetes is the diabetes that has its onset during pregnancy and goes away after pregnancy. Secondary diabetes is that diabetes resulting from another disease. Once the other disease is cured, then the diabetes goes away. Classic examples of secondary diabetes include Cushing's disease (a disease characterized by too much cortisol, a hormone made in the adrenal gland), acromegaly (giantism), and pheochromocytoma (a vascular tumor of the adrenal medulla).

It's important that not only the diagnosis of diabetes be made but also the correct classification in order to help guide the best therapy to normalize the high glucose levels. Type I diabetic persons require insulin therapy; Type II diabetic persons may do well on diet, exercise, and/or oral agents (blood-sugar-lowering pills).

JUNE AND BARBARA: Are the symptoms of Type I and Type II diabetes different?

DR. LOIS: Yes. When a person develops Type I diabetes, the effects of hyperglycemia (high blood sugar) are manifest immediately: great thirst and urination, constant hunger, massive weight loss, and irritability. If the diabetes isn't treated with immediate insulin therapy, the irritability will turn to disorientation, coma, and eventual death.

Type II diabetes creeps up gradually, and symptoms are therefore tolerated. A person may not be bothered by the high blood sugars until these high blood-glucose levels cause other problems, like vaginitis or foot infections. These symptoms confirm the diagnosis but are not necessary to it.

JUNE AND BARBARA: June's symptoms were that subtle kind. She, who was normally healthy to a fault, kept getting sore throats and colds that lingered and lingered. Incidentally, because her symptoms were gradual and because she was forty-five when her diabetes was diagnosed, we think of her as a Type II. And yet she did have to go on insulin. We have a theory, based strictly on observation, that the Type IIs who are thin generally have to go on insulin, while the overweight ones can often control their diabetes through diet, exercise, and sometimes pills after losing their excess weight. We've heard that the French categorize diabetics as *"maigres"* (thins) and *"gras"* (fats) rather than as Type I and Type II. Their belief is that the *maigres* usually have to go on insulin and that the *gras* usually don't. Do you agree with this?

DR. LOIS: Yes, I agree, although some Type IIs are really Type Is who are on their way to complete pancreatic "poopout" and thus need insulin all along. Other thin Type IIs *are* really thin Type IIs, and with rigorous exercise, a low-carbohydrate diet, and the oral hypoglycemic agents, they can squeak by without insulin. But insulin is the best treatment for the majority of thin Type IIs.

Fat Type IIs have plenty of insulin coming from their pancreases. Their problem is that they cannot clear the sugar after it is eaten. The treatment of choice for them is to restrict their amount of food so that the sugar does not build up in the bloodstream.

JUNE AND BARBARA: A woman who got "instant diabetes" from having 85 percent of her pancreas removed complained to us that her surgeon and family doctor disagree on the long-term outlook, and she can find no information on this form of diabetes. Could you, as they say, compare and contrast (as they like to put it on college essay examinations) surgically induced diabetes with the standard variety?

DR. LOIS: Sometimes surgical removal of the pancreas (pancreatectomy) is necessary in the case of pancreatic carcinoma, insulinomas, and certain forms of pancreatitis (infectious), specifically, idiopathic (of unknown cause) and/or alcoholic pancreatitis. In these cases, when the pancreas is removed all of the pancreatic functions are removed, not just the insulin-producing cells. The pancreas also makes digestive enzymes. When these are removed, the result is a malabsorption syndrome. This syndrome includes protein and fat wasting, plus deficiencies of vitamins A, D, E, and K because these vitamins are absorbed with fat in the gut. In addition, glucagon, the hormone that raises blood sugar, which is produced by the alpha cells in the pancreas, is missing. Thus, this diabetes is difficult to manage for many reasons.

The insulin requirement is usually one-half to two-thirds less for a person whose pancreas has been removed than for a Type I diabetic person, since without glucagon there is not the usual buffer against insulin action. These patients can go into DKA (diabetic ketoacidosis), despite the old teaching that DKA is associated with elevated glucagon levels. These people prove that DKA is the result of absolute insulin lack.

People whose pancreases have been surgically removed are exquisitely brittle (unstable). They can go very low with a low dose of insulin, because the food they eat does not get into their bloodstream due to the lack of digestive enzymes.

JUNE AND BARBARA: Sometimes when people are first diagnosed as having diabetes they race to a dictionary or encyclopedia and by mistake read about diabetes insipidus, which has nothing to do with their condition. To alleviate this confusion could you explain what that other disease, diabetes insipidus, is?

**DR. LOIS:** Diabetes insipidus is also a disease characterized by massive urination. The cause of this urination, however, is a lack of a hormone called vasopressin or antidiuretic hormone. The posterior pituitary gland makes this hormone, and if a tumor destroys the posterior pituitary, water is spontaneously lost from the kidneys.

**JUNE AND BARBARA:** We've always understood that more women than men have diabetes, but at the ADA (American Diabetes Association) Conference where we heard you speak, we also heard a talk at which it was pointed out that in Europe men are now in the majority.

**DR. LOIS:** For Type I diabetics, it's usually fifty-fifty, but at times it changes to forty-sixty or sixty-forty. It's like the gender swings in baby booms.

For Type II it's more likely to be 65 to 70 percent women and 30 to 35 percent men.

**JUNE AND BARBARA:** Why us?

**DR. LOIS:** Women have more body fat than men, even in the normal weight range (25 to 30 percent in women versus 18 to 25 percent in men). Increased body fat increases your chances for diabetes when the heredity is there. In the abnormal ranges, women tend to be more obese than men. They also tend to gain weight during pregnancy, and this weight is often not entirely shed afterward.

There is also the factor that Type II diabetes is inherited more from the mother's side than from the father's side.

JUNE AND BARBARA: One diabetic sociologist of our acquaintance maintains that women have more diabetes than men because of the stresses of being pulled in every direction, trying to fill every role that society seems to require of them: housekeeper, gourmet cook, lover and companion to her husband, mother, career woman, etc. She says that no matter what a woman is doing at a given moment, she feels guilty because she's not doing something else. Do you think those stresses could be a factor in bringing out diabetes?

DR. LOIS: Of course, if you try to be a superwoman, that's going to create stress, and stress does bring out and exacerbate diabetes. I once heard of an organization in San Francisco called "Superwomen Anonymous," founded by Carol Orsborn, author of *Enough Is Enough: Exploding the Myth of Having It All.* This organization is geared toward helping women who are caught up in trying to have it all. Maybe joining that would be a help for stressed-out diabetic women. But stress isn't exclusive to the female sex. Some of my male patients double their insulin requirement during the week of April 15. It's more a matter of the individual and her or his ability to cope with the stresses that assail everyone in modern society.

JUNE AND BARBARA: Yes, coping is the key. You know, way back in 1980 we wrote an entire book, *The Diabetic's Total Health Book* (revised in 1992), focusing on the role of stress in diabetes. Because of June's personal experience and stories we heard from other diabetics, we saw the devastating effects of the stressors of contemporary life on chronic health problems such as diabetes. We presented in that book a smorgasbord of relaxation therapies, beginning with biofeedback technique and continuing with progressive relaxation, autogenic training, meditation, guided imagery, and such unorthodox methods as laughter and hug therapy. All of these techniques work if you practice them regularly. You just have to discover which ones work best for you and then—here's the crucial factor—take or make time to do them.

DR. LOIS: We advised patients in a study we did [published in *Diabetes Care*, November–December 1985] to use biofeedback relaxation twice a day and whenever a difficult situation arose in their lives. We did learn one exception to the effectiveness of stress reduction therapies. None of our patients could control their blood-sugar levels in times of catastrophic events. We learned that when something really traumatic happens—death of a loved one, car accident, robbery, fire, school failure, etc.—it is normal to forget diabetes self-care and relaxation techniques. The crisis takes precedence, making it impossible to think of anything but the disaster itself. Therefore, it is best to cope with the disaster and avoid feeling guilty about transient loss of diabetes control. Then, when the crisis has passed, diabetes control can take center stage once more.

JUNE AND BARBARA: A number of people would put you in the superwoman category, since you are a physician, wife, and mother, along with your many other roles. Do you find that when you're under heavy stress, your blood sugars tend to go up and/or you need to increase your insulin?

DR. LOIS: Yes, I do wax and wane when stress appears, but my eating habits tend to change when I am under stress, so it's hard to figure out entirely. I must say that my insulin requirement has dropped 10 percent now that

I'm a "laid back" Californian instead of a high-powered New Yorker. This decreased insulin requirement is even more amazing because I have also gained weight. I guess stress did contribute a bit to my overall control.

In our biofeedback relaxation study, relaxation exercises did decrease the insulin requirement and improve the instability of glucose levels up to 20 percent in selected patients.

Incidentally, many diabetics don't realize that diabetes is itself a great stress factor. You have to worry about high and low blood sugars and you have to remember to have food along wherever you go, as well as your insulin and testing materials. Diabetes is always there in the back of your mind, and that builds up the stress level.

**JUNE AND BARBARA:** In a letter we received, a woman pointed out that there are both advantages and disadvantages to being a diabetic woman rather than a diabetic man. Her theory was that women have an advantage because they generally understand food better and also that they can make a better psychological adjustment to the disease because they don't have to present a tough macho image, which might make men ashamed to wear a pump or do something else that would help their control. On the other hand, she felt that women had a disadvantage in that it's usually hard for them to put themselves first, and as a result their diabetes is generally more unstable. Do you agree with her "good news, bad news" theory?

**DR. LOIS:** Not entirely. I can't really think of why it might be an advantage to be a diabetic woman rather than a diabetic man. Women don't necessarily understand food. They know taste, quality, texture, color, freshness, and so forth. The nutrient value of food is not the main topic in Julia Child's gourmet cooking class. Both men and women take health class in junior high school, and it's as easy for a man to memorize food values as a woman. A man may not be in charge of the food he eats, but why should a man be in poor diabetic control because his wife seasons with sugar or honey? He could investigate the problem and solve it as well as a woman.

Now that the pumps are small enough to be easily hidden in a pocket, the issue of publicly wearing your diabetes is no longer a valid issue, macho feelings or not.

It's true, however, that the menstrual cycle changes the insulin requirement. The insulin therefore needs adjusting once a month for women, whereas men are pretty stable except during times of business stress, when the blood-glucose level can increase by two or three times. Also, pregnancy is a lot more complicated for a woman with diabetes than for a man with diabetes!

I must admit, too, that it's often difficult for a woman to put herself first, since she's so accustomed to taking care of everyone else in the family.

JUNE AND BARBARA: That's certainly true. We've noticed that it's often hard for a woman to take the time out to care for herself when she has a cold, let alone when she has something as time-consuming and inexorable as diabetes. We always maintain that you must take care of yourself or you won't be able to do anything for others.

If you aren't willing to make the effort to control your diabetes for yourself, how about doing it for those you love? In that way you can free them from worrying about your diabetes and allow them to live up to their fullest potential. The following note, which came attached to an announcement of the writer's graduation from law school, shows how very important your control can be to others. Although it's from a woman writing about her diabetic husband, it holds true for either sex.

> Dear June and Barbara:
> We purchased a meter in December. Since then my husband's diabetes has been controlled. It certainly took a load of worry off my mind during my last year in law school. In that light I wanted to share my graduation with you. Thanks for all your help!

One young woman confessed to us that her husband had told her that she used to be disagreeable about half the time—"a real bitch" was how he put it. But since she had started controlling her blood sugar, "she's become a wonderful human being and a joy to be around."

And while you're controlling your blood sugar for the benefit of others, you should start investigating why you don't control it for yourself. Don't you consider yourself important? Aren't you worth the effort? Don't you love yourself enough?

To return from psychology to physiology, one woman wrote to ask if more women than men are affected by diabetic neuropathy. The reason she asked was that many Type II diabetic women in her diabetes group developed neuropathy but none of the men did (although, she pointed out, men rarely attended the meetings).

DR. LOIS: Type II diabetes is more common among women than men, so naturally more of them would develop neuropathy. But if the question is asked about Type I diabetics, men get neuropathy just as frequently as women.

JUNE AND BARBARA: We think this is a rather minor controversy, but some otherwise rational people get quite shrill about it. Do you have any strong opinion, based on either your own feelings or those reported to you by your patients, about whether a person should say "I am a diabetic" or "I have diabetes"? June doesn't care one way or the other, but she usually says the former. Exponents of the "I have diabetes" school maintain that their diabetes is only a secondary consideration and feel that if they say "I am a diabetic," it intrudes on the dignity of their personhood.

DR. LOIS: Funny, I think the only people who are fussy about this are nondiabetics. I always say that it doesn't matter if I am a person with syphilis or if I am a syphilitic—I still have the same disease. Actually, it is incorrect to use the word *diabetic* as a noun, and the American Diabetes Association will not allow its use in this way. In the final analysis, I'm not particularly happy with any label.

JUNE AND BARBARA: Enough of these nomenclatural shenanigans. Whether you call yourself a woman diabetic or a diabetic woman, what is the best type of doctor to see? An internist? A gynecologist? A diabetologist? An endocrinologist?

DR. LOIS: Ideally, every diabetic woman should have the luxury of three doctors—a diabetologist, an internist, and a gynecologist—and one dentist.

However, depending on what area of the country she lives in and on her finances, a diabetic woman may be able to choose only one doctor. A well-trained internist should be able to adjust insulin or oral hypoglycemic agents, do Pap smears, and treat other ailments, too. But an internist often does not have adequate time, teaching materials, or support staff for intensive diabetes management. Thus, if a diabetic woman wants an intensified management program, she may be disappointed with the minimal interaction she may get related to diabetes issues.

JUNE AND BARBARA: Incidentally, many people, ourselves included, are confused by the terms used for physicians specializing in diabetes. Many are called endocrinologists and others diabetologists. Are they the same?

DR. LOIS: They *can* be the same, but they aren't always. Let me explain: an endocrinologist is board certified in that specialty by the American College of Physicians; a diabetologist is any physician who specializes in the treatment of diabetes and who mainly treats diabetics. An internist or general practitioner could be a diabetologist, as could an endocrinologist who specializes in diabetes.

JUNE AND BARBARA: Going to the doctor seems to be stressful for everyone. Women (and men) like to tell us war stories about their doctors. Some of the doctors are portrayed as saints, but to be honest, a good percentage of the time he or she is made to sound like an avaricious devil who gives virtually no attention to the patient's problems. And we see the other side, too—patients who seem to feel that the doctor has an obligation to them, to the exclusion of all other patients, to give them infinite time for even the most infinitesimal complaints and to then charge only a token amount for their services.

It reminds us of when we were librarians in the Los Angeles Community College District. One of our colleagues wryly remarked, "The professors think they should be paid for staying at home, and the district thinks they should work for nothing." The answer has to lie somewhere in between. So must it lie somewhere in between for patients and doctors.

As a physician and a diabetic woman, you can see both sides of the picture. Could you give us an idea of what a diabetic patient has a legitimate right to expect from a doctor's visit?

DR. LOIS: It also has something to do with being a woman as well as a diabetic. Women of necessity visit physicians more than men do. We're locked into a compulsory visit to the gynecologist for a Pap smear, and when we have babies numerous doctor visits are necessary.

Let's examine the case of a doctor's visit for a Pap smear. Although the purpose of this visit is to have a simple test, somehow we feel cheated if the doctor doesn't take time to talk to us and show concern. Thus, our expectations of what we think the purpose of this visit is are clearly different from what the doctor thinks the purpose of this visit is.

On top of a background of preconceived expectations, a diabetic woman visits a diabetes specialist. I shall now take the point of view of a physician and describe what I think should happen in the doctor's office, and then I'll describe my response as a diabetic woman who is given this care.

At the initial visit the doctor should take a complete history, including the following points:

Age
Duration of diabetes
Medications

Insulin history (a review of types of insulin and number of injections along with dosages and needs, especially if the times of the doses have significantly changed)

Number of episodes of ketoacidosis and need for hospitalizations

Number of severe hypoglycemia episodes and review of the most recent history of even minor hypoglycemia

Assessment of control—type of glucose monitoring done and typical patterns over the years

History of complications of diabetes, specifically those related to the eyes, kidneys, feet, and nerves

Menstrual history—onset, frequency, character, and duration

Pregnancy-related history

Family history, not only of diabetes but also of heart disease, hypertension, and seizure disorders

Other coexisting illnesses

Previous surgery

History of allergies

History of severe infections: ear, pneumonia, urine, and/or kidney

Then the doctor should ask the patient the reason for the visit. Is it just a checkup? Does the patient want a change in insulin dosage? Is the patient seeking better control? Does the patient have a complication of diabetes that she is worried about? Based on the chief reason for the visit, the doctor will then direct more questions toward trying to come to an answer to the problems. The total time to take the history should be about fifteen to twenty minutes.

The initial visit should also include a complete physical examination, but one that's directed to diabetes-related problems:

Height, weight, blood pressure, pulse

Eyes: the back of the eye will be examined.

Nose, ears, mouth, tongue, teeth, and skin

Neck: emphasis on thyroid and lymph glands

Chest: the doctor will listen with the stethoscope to both lungs and heart.

Abdomen: the doctor will check here for liver, spleen, and enlarged uterus and will listen with the stethoscope for bowel sounds and abnormal blood-vessel noises.

Groin area: pulses and lymph glands

Pelvic and rectal: the diabetes doctor will usually not do a pelvic or rectal examination but rather will confirm with the patient that she does have a gynecologist.

Legs and feet: these will be examined for pulses, muscle strength, and nerve function, including ankle and knee jerks and sensation and position sense.

The total time for the complete physical examination should be around twenty to thirty minutes.

Based on the history and the physical, the doctor will formulate a problem list and a plan of attack. The patient will be asked to get dressed and then meet the doctor in the consultation room to learn about her problems and the possible solutions to them.

Let's assume that the patient came to the diabetes specialist for improvement of blood-sugar control and that she was well, with no complications of diabetes. The doctor would then first reinforce good preventive-care habits, including such basics as an eye-doctor appointment at least once a year, care with cutting toenails, etc.

The doctor would then set up a series of follow-up appointments to see that any suggested change in insulin dose meets the needs of the patient and to discuss the results of laboratory tests ordered. The essential laboratory tests include glycosylated hemoglobin (see related question later in this chapter), thyroid-function tests, kidney tests, blood count, and blood-chemistry tests.

Like the history and the physical, this discussion period should last from twenty to thirty minutes. Note that the doctor can by no means prescribe a "better" dose of insulin in this session. Instead, a stepwise plan should be created that includes education on diet, exercise, home blood-glucose monitoring, charting, sick-day procedures, and the like. Most of the educational interaction will be between the patient and the nurse and/or dietitian. Subsequent visits to the nurse and dietitian will probably be made when the doctor may not be available. Phone contact will likely be through the office nurse and may not be directly to the physician.

Once a patient's new diabetes program is under way (establishing a new program may take several closely spaced visits), a repeat visit should occur three to four times a year for checkup and laboratory blood tests. Each of these visits will be around twenty to thirty minutes long.

Now, how do I as a patient respond to the treatment described above? It depends on my expectations. If I thought the doctor was going to be my only health-care professional, I might resent the nurse and/or dietitian, although these people usually are better teachers than a busy doctor. Perhaps I came in for one visit to have my blood sugars fixed and found that my doctor couldn't give me a magic dose of insulin in one visit but insisted that I come back several times to visit his nurse, keep tedious records of my own blood tests, and stick to a rigid diet. On top of all the work that I was assigned, I was billed for each and every visit, even if I did not see the doctor. Never mind that my blood-sugar level improved.

Rather than experience a series of disappointments, it would be better to begin the first visit by telling the doctor what you expect and then having the doctor tell you what will happen. Then, with agreement, you and the doctor can problem-solve together.

JUNE AND BARBARA: That covers the physiological aspects of a diabetic woman's visit to the doctor. Now, how about the emotional aspects? Could you imagine for us that you're in the office with a Type I diabetic woman who is either newly diagnosed or who has had diabetes for a year or less?

DR. LOIS: It's not hard for me to imagine this scene, since I've often had the occasion to consult with patients within a year of their diagnosis. Unfortunately, I find that as a whole the health-professional community hasn't met the needs of a woman who is given the diagnosis of a chronic disease at a young age.

Just as there are five stages of grieving when a person loses a loved one, there are five stages of grieving when a person is confronted with the diagnosis of diabetes. Stage one is disbelief and denial. Much of this stage is spent arguing with the Almighty and negotiating a reprieve. Stage two is anger. Why me? Stage three is depression and withdrawal. Stage four is recovery, and stage five is acceptance. It usually takes a year to complete the entire process of grief.

I usually meet the women during their depression. They are even more depressed because their previous doctor usually hasn't allowed such indulgence in "self-pity." They get reprimands and rejection from their doctors instead of the support they so desperately need. This intensifies their depression.

Nothing seems to help more than my telling these women that a year for the entire grief process is the norm and that some people take longer. This rids them of false feelings of guilt or of the conviction that their behavior is weak or aberrant.

I've also often heard from patients that they have been told their diabetes is too mild for an intensive program of care. As a result, they're given no education about the rationale for controlling blood sugar or about how it is to be achieved. They're not even asked if they prefer an intensive program.

The last, and probably the worst, problem is the fear these women have about asking simple questions that emerge from the soul. Will I be frigid? Lose my legs? Be blind and die on a kidney machine? These are very real fears for a woman who has read about diabetes in the women's magazines before she knew that one day she would develop the disease. Merely telling patients that most complications of diabetes do not happen for five to ten years after the diagnosis is a relief to most newly diagnosed persons. Then a teachable moment is reached in which I can make a plug for good glucose control to reinforce that the woman is keeper of her own fate and that she does not have to be a victim of her own disease.

It would be unfair to the woman, however, if I didn't admit to her that there are a few problems that do happen immediately. High blood sugar increases anxiety and irritability and requires greater coping skills. I can assure her, though, that the unstable personality she's now experiencing can be helped by stabilizing her blood-sugar levels. Better blood sugar can also help any uncomfortable vaginitis she may be experiencing. It's worth it for me to adjust a patient's therapy to alleviate these two problems alone, even if it means more than one injection a day of insulin.

**JUNE AND BARBARA:** We've noticed that diabetic women tend to blame every physical problem they have—from dandruff to hangnails—on their diabetes. Are there certain conditions in which a woman is justified in accusing her diabetes?

**DR. LOIS:** Let's not say diabetes, but *out-of-control* diabetes. There's a vast difference between the two. Well-controlled diabetes is usually innocent until proven guilty, but out-of-control diabetes could well be a prime suspect in the following:

1. Vaginitis, specifically fungal in origin
2. Staphylococcal infections of the skin, such as boils, impetigo, and abscesses
3. Depression in states of both severe hyperglycemia and hypoglycemia
4. Changes of refractive error of the lens so that your glasses always seem too weak
5. Headaches (from hypoglycemia)
6. Insomnia and/or nightmares (from hypoglycemia)
7. Menstrual irregularities
8. Gum disease, which may lead to premature loss of teeth
9. High blood lipids (cholesterol, triglycerides)
10. Hypertension (high blood pressure)
11. Anemia
12. Decaying nails, specifically toenails
13. Necrobiosis diabeticorum (shin spots)
14. Osteoporosis (brittle bones)

15. Easy exhaustion from exercise or inability to achieve a training response to exercise. (Hyperglycemia does not let a muscle work; lactic acid builds up, and the pain prevents the person from continuing with the exercise. This stress causes the blood sugar to continue to rise and sets up a vicious cycle.)
16. Cataracts
17. Salivary-gland stones

JUNE AND BARBARA: That's a long list of reasons to keep diabetes in control. Are there some other conditions that could be related to diabetes but that generally are not?

DR. LOIS: That list is equally long, and it includes these conditions:

1. Itching
2. Headaches
3. Sinusitis
4. Vertigo
5. Tinnitus (a ringing in the ears)
6. Dizziness
7. Certain lung infections, including tuberculosis
8. Heart attacks
9. Gall-bladder disease and stones
10. Kidney and urine infections
11. Infertility
12. Hirsutism (excessive body and facial hair)
13. Amenorrhea (failure to menstruate)
14. Delayed puberty
15. Short stature
16. Contraction of joints
17. Neuropathy (more common from ingesting too much alcohol than from diabetes-related causes)

JUNE AND BARBARA: If we ruled the world, even if we couldn't eliminate disease entirely, we'd at least make it only one to a customer. In other words, if you had one disease you couldn't get another. Is this rule already in effect in any way with diabetes? Is there any disease you're less likely to have if you have diabetes?

DR. LOIS: Unfortunately, not to any extent. The only diseases I can think of that are less likely in diabetic women than in nondiabetic women are lupus erythematosus and sickle-cell anemia.

JUNE AND BARBARA: Well, at least that's something. But let's go back to that point you made about the vast difference between in-control diabetes and out-of-control diabetes. Unfortunately, not all physicians make that distinction. When we were speaking at a diabetes conference at the Eisenhower Medical Center in Palm Desert, we listened to the physician speakers to learn more, as we always do. And as always, we heard again and again the dismal statistics about people with diabetes—how they're this percentage more likely to go blind and that percentage more likely to have kidney failure and the other percentage more likely to have one or more feet amputated.

June looked over at diabetic triathlete Bill Carlson, who was also in the audience. He was lean and fit and glowing with health. He'd been on a bike ride of 110 miles the day before and on his usual long-distance run that morning. What did these statistics have to do with him? And June considered herself and the fact that at her age she was in much better shape than all of her nondiabetic contemporaries and many of those ten or fifteen years younger. Her blood sugars were better than ever. (Practice makes perfect—well, *almost* perfect.) What did these statistics have to do with her? At dinner that night we discussed this situation. June theorized that there should now be two new categories of diabetes classification: Type C (for controlled) and Type U (for uncontrolled). They're really two different diseases with two different prognoses.

The fact that the dismal statistics of the past dealt with Type U diabetics only was proven in 1993 with the completion of the Diabetes Control and Complications Trial (DCCT), a ten-year U.S. government study involving 1,441 Type I diabetics. Half the participants were on the old conventional therapy—one or two shots of insulin a day and one blood-sugar test—and half were on an "intensive treatment" of a minimum of four blood-sugar tests a day and three or four shots of insulin or an insulin pump. Those on intensive treatment were also required to adjust insulin doses according to food intake and exercise. Even though the intensive control group had blood-sugar levels somewhat above those of nondiabetics, they were much closer to normal than those using conventional therapy.

The DCCT results were convincing, even to previous skeptics. Diabetic retinopathy was reduced by 76 percent, kidney disease was prevented or delayed by 56 percent, and neuropathy (nerve damage) by 60 percent. Though this study was limited to Type I diabetes, the American Diabetes Association in their Position Statement conclude that it seems reasonable to recommend tight control in many Type II patients, since it is presumed that the cause of complications would be the same in both types. A planned similar study for Type II is expected to confirm that logical conclusion.

Our idea is that we should all work toward that happy day when every diabetic is either a Type IC or a Type IIC, with not a Type U to be seen. In pursuit of that goal, maybe you could tell us the control that we should shoot for (pun intended). We find that many of the diabetics we talk to—even some long-term diabetics—don't really know what their blood sugars should be. What constitutes the happy-medium condition known as euglycemia—not too high, not too low, but, like the baby bear's bed in the story of Goldilocks, just right?

DR. LOIS: The answer to that is that the fasting or premeal blood sugar should be between 70 and 100; one hour after a meal, it should be 140; and two hours after a meal, it should be 120.

To achieve these blood sugars, which average 100 mg/dl, we allow the "swing" room to be down to 50 and up to 150, swinging around 100. This doesn't mean that we wouldn't decrease the insulin if the blood sugar were 50, but in the overall picture we accept these extremes.

JUNE AND BARBARA: Do blood sugars vary from age to age? For example, are normal blood sugars for children different from normal blood sugars for adults?

DR. LOIS: Yes, blood-sugar levels do vary with age. A newborn has a normal blood sugar of 40 to 60 mg/dl. Children ages one through five usually have fasting blood sugars of 60 mg/dl. Then, from eight to thirty years it stays at 70. After thirty years the fasting blood sugar goes up 1 mg/dl per year. So twenty years later, at the age of fifty, the normal fasting blood sugar is around 100 mg/dl. By the age of eighty, it may go to 130 mg/dl. This is all to say that the normal pancreas ages, and that as it does it gradually loses function.

JUNE AND BARBARA: No matter what your age, of course, you want to be in good control. In order to achieve this goal, most of you have to know what your blood sugars are every day—in fact, for intensive therapy several times a day. Therefore, you have to be testing your blood sugar yourself.

Ever since it came on the scene, we've been passionate advocates of self-testing for blood sugar. June was doing it way back in 1978, when the only meter was the Ames Eyetone reflectance meter. The reason she got so excited about blood-sugar testing was that with the urine tests of that era she always looked as if she were doing just fine, but when she started testing her blood sugar she was amazed and aghast to discover that even when her urine tests said she was normal, her blood sugar could be well over 200. Like many diabetic women over forty, she has a high renal threshold. This means that her kidneys don't spill sugar into her urine until her blood sugar is quite high, so according to the urine tests everything looked normal. Although in those days a meter cost $650, June was determined to get one, because she knew it was the only way to know what was really happening to her blood sugar. (Luckily, she was able to find a used one for a reasonable price.)

June attributes the fact that she has absolutely no complications after twenty-eight years of diabetes to two strategies: testing her blood sugar six or seven times a day, and taking five shots of insulin a day plus supplements when her blood sugar is not normal. Do you feel as strongly as we do about the advantages of blood-sugar testing over urine testing?

**DR. LOIS:** Absolutely. In explaining the difference between urine testing and blood-sugar testing to my patients, I like to use this automobile-speedometer analogy: Suppose you owned a car with a speedometer that was always way behind your actual driving speed—

say, it would read thirty when you were actually going sixty miles an hour. Let's also say that the penalty for driving at sixty was life in prison. What would you do? You would surely get a new speedometer.

Such a lagging speedometer can be compared to testing your urine for sugar, when what you really need to know is the amount of sugar in your *blood* at any given moment. The sugar in your urine merely tells you about the sugar that was in your blood hours ago. Too late to prevent an arrest!

JUNE AND BARBARA: Nevertheless, we still hear of physicians who have their patients test their urine along with their blood sugar. Do you feel there's any necessity for this?

DR. LOIS: I usually don't play up urine tests, because I feel it distracts patients from blood-sugar tests. The only urine test I usually recommend is for ketones, which are substances formed during the metabolism of fat. When blood sugars are excessively high, the body converts its own fat into fuel. Ketones are released from fat cells when the cells break down from not having enough insulin in the bloodstream to hold them together. There are three fatty acids that are released from the fat cell. These three acids go to the liver, which converts them to ketones. A buildup of ketones makes the blood dangerously acidic.

JUNE AND BARBARA: When is it important to test for ketones?

DR. LOIS: I recommend it when the blood sugar is over 250.

**JUNE AND BARBARA:** What should you do if you find you have ketones?

**DR. LOIS:** Add one unit of regular insulin for every 25 mg/dl you are above 250. For instance, if you are 400 and there are ketones in your urine, take six units of regular insulin. Drink lots of water, and call the physician for further advice.

**JUNE AND BARBARA:** Another important test for assaying your control is the glycosylated-hemoglobin, or hemoglobin $A_{1C}$ test. Many women haven't heard of this at all and others have only a vague idea of what it is, of who needs it, and of what the results should be. Can you help us with that?

**DR. LOIS:** In the early sixties a blood banker noted that 5 percent of the donors had an elevation of a component of hemoglobin that was barely present in the other 95 percent of the population. He then noted that these individuals were the same persons who had diabetes. He concluded from this that there is a genetic marker for diabetes. It was not until the mid-seventies that it was learned that it is the sugar in the blood of diabetic persons that modifies hemoglobin to $A_{1C}$ and not diabetes *per se*.

Thus, hemoglobin $A_{1C}$ is a modified component of hemoglobin A (which is the majority of hemoglobin in our blood). The higher the blood-glucose level, the more hemoglobin A becomes hemoglobin $A_{1C}$. The reaction is essentially irreversible, and once hemoglobin $A_{1C}$ is formed it stays formed for the life span of the red-blood cell (about 120 days).

The formula is: hemoglobin A + sugar yields hemoglobin $A_{1C}$.

The hemoglobin $A_{1C}$ test can be used as a retrospect scope in that the amount of hemoglobin $A_{1C}$ is directly related to the glucose levels over time. While the on rate for sugar onto hemoglobin A is rapid, the off rate is slow. In other words, it is more sensitive to sin than to repentance. The on rate is one to two weeks of high blood-glucose levels; the off rate is six weeks to two months.

The test is simple in that it does not require the woman to be fasting, since it is not affected by the moment-to-moment variations of blood glucose. Neither is it very sensitive to minor changes in blood glucose: in order for the hemoglobin $A_{1C}$ to be raised by 1 percent, the blood-sugar average needs to be 20 mg/dl higher. The normal range varies from laboratory to laboratory. Thus, a woman should not only ask what the result of her test is but also what is normal for the particular laboratory.

Glycosylated hemoglobin cannot be used to make the diagnosis of diabetes, as it is not sensitive enough. This diagnosis can only be made through a glucose-tolerance test.

As a monitor of glucose levels over time, an $A_{1C}$ is good for about two months. Therefore, as a double check on a woman's diabetes program, $A_{1C}$ tests should be taken no farther apart than every three months. This frequency in checking allows for intervention before prolonged periods of high blood-glucose levels take their toll.

JUNE AND BARBARA: A woman who had a rather dismal experience with her diabetes while in the hospital wants to know what you can do to maintain your control when the nurses and doctors take over and seem to be making your blood sugars bounce around in a very scary way, not to mention the fact that the food that arrives on your tray is often too much of the wrong thing. In fact, we constantly hear stories from experienced diabetic women about traumatic hospital stays.

DR. LOIS: What happens is that education is a blessing in disguise, for the more you know, the more frustrating it is to be treated inappropriately. All of my well-educated patients find themselves in situations in which they know more than the health-care team. There are several positive results of this potentially anxiety-provoking situation. First, become a gentle teacher and explain that you measure your own blood sugar and that it helps you to decide your own doses of insulin. Consequently, you need access to your meter and insulin. The physician in charge should be able to help you get permission to continue to do self-care, even though you are in a hospital.

Second, allow the staff to test your meter if they are not sure of its accuracy. They want to see how close you can get to the lab result. If you can accurately measure your sugar, you have proven that you can use your meter skillfully, and this demonstration will usually stop the blood-drawing team from sticking you!

Third, if things are not exactly the way you want, allow for a bit of flexibility. Usually their way is not so bad.

Finally, above all remember that you still have rights as a citizen and can refuse anything that does not seem right.

As far as my own stories go, it is amazing to me that I have had the dumb luck of consistent mishaps. But it doesn't happen just to me. My six-year-old daughter was in the hospital to have an orthopedic procedure performed on her left leg. The surgeon came by and picked up her right leg and said, "We'll have this leg perfect again in the morning." My daughter told him that her right leg was perfect and she wanted her *left* leg fixed! I was so worried that I wrote "Fix this one" across her left leg as they took her off to the operating room. The moral of the story is that you should be assertive—if something is not right, speak out!

JUNE AND BARBARA: We received a letter containing a specific question that may actually turn out to be a more general one: "About eleven years after developing diabetes, I developed a thyroid condition known as Graves' disease. My doctor did not think it was related to my diabetes, but a year later I read an article in the *ADA Forecast* that said that thyroid conditions do seem to be somehow related to diabetes. Do women seem more prone to this than men?"

DR. LOIS: Forty percent of all Type I patients have a coexisting thyroid disease. This is presumably based on the same antibody attack on the thyroid as on the pancreas. Other glands that can also be attacked are the adrenal, ovary, pituitary, and parathyroids, as well as the stomach lining, which produces $B_{12}$. For this reason all diabetic women should be checked periodically for the status of these glands.

JUNE AND BARBARA: Some women have complained about leg cramps. Do you know what causes these and what they can do about them?

DR. LOIS: Leg cramps tend to happen to all people, men or women, diabetic persons or nondiabetic persons. However, with large swings in blood glucose, other ions such as sodium, potassium, and calcium, which because of their chemical properties of positive charge are called *cations,* also tend to swing. Leg cramps are the result of these cationic fluxes. The blood levels of these cations do not reflect their muscle levels. There are many causes of cationic disturbances at the muscle level, among them:

> chronic diuretic therapy with muscle potassium loss,
> extremes of calcium intake—too little for a long time or too much for a long time—and
> stasis, which can be caused by sitting too long, wearing high boots or knee-high hose, having varicose veins, or being pregnant (which can stop the blood return from the legs).

The best treatment is to replace potassium losses, normalize calcium intake, avoid wearing knee-highs or high boots, avoid sitting for longer than an hour without raising the legs, give birth, and—last but not least—do stretching exercises before bed. If the muscle is stretched before bed, it will have less of a tendency to cramp up. My favorite exercise is to stand four to five feet from the wall and then lean into it, holding the position while I watch the 11 P.M. news.

JUNE AND BARBARA: We had an inquiry from a woman in her forties, an artist and photographer who does quite strenuous gymnastics. She wanted to know about microalbumin—specifically, why it appears in the urine after heavy workouts and whether it leads to kidney disease.

DR. LOIS: Exercise increases cardiac output. As the blood rushes past the kidney, albumin—a small molecular-weight protein—is filtered into the urine. Albumin usually does not appear in the urine unless the pressure is increased, as is the case with strenuous exercise. Microalbuminuria, or albumin in the urine, is a normal response to strenuous exercise. Albumin is also lost when the kidney has been damaged because of diabetes, causing the filter to become "leaky." Although both situations produce albumin in the urine, exercise does not increase the leak from diabetic nephropathy.

JUNE AND BARBARA: Apparently her gymnastics aren't doing her any harm, then, and that's great assurance. We hope every woman will have *some* kind of exercise program worked into her life. Surely everyone can squeeze in at least five days weekly of a thirty-minute session (okay, a twenty-minute session if you have to). This can be fifteen minutes of strength training with weights or Nautilus-type machines and fifteen minutes of aerobic activity. The strength-training segment is really important, because you get maximum gain for minimum time plus better body shaping and more muscle. Now hear this: Muscles burn more calories than fat; therefore, muscle building is good for weight loss.

The reason we're coming on so strong about exercise is that we have long been fanatics about its health and blood-sugar control benefits. In fact, recently in collaboration with Claudia Graham, a diabetic who has a Ph.D. in Exercise Science, we updated our *The Diabetes Sports and Exercise Book*. That's where you can find all the details of an exercise program, whatever your age or current physical condition.

Dr. Lois, lest we go overboard with our enthusiasm, can you give us some sports and exercise precautions?

DR. LOIS: Yes, women with retinopathy should avoid any exercise that places the head below the heart, because it is thought that this increased pressure in the eye can lead to bleeding in the retina.

JUNE AND BARBARA: Would weight-lifting and/or strenuous high-impact aerobic dancing also be bad for someone with retinopathy?

DR. LOIS: Yes, this too would raise pressure in the eye. Consult with your eye doctor if you have retinopathy so that he or she can help you plan a safe exercise program.

Of course, a diabetic woman should check her blood sugar before any exercise session to ensure that she does not have a hypoglycemic episode during the session. A well-controlled woman should exercise with her blood glucose at 70 to 150 mg/dl and should check her blood sugar every twenty minutes to make sure it isn't dropping.

JUNE AND BARBARA: She also needs to have some idea of how much carbohydrate that exercise is going to burn in order to prevent low blood sugar with a preexercise snack. We use a handy chart created by John Walsh for his booklet, *The Pocket Pancreas.* It is reprinted below:

### Grams of Carbohydrate Used per Hour in Different Exercises

| Activity | Your Weight: | | |
| | 100 lb | 150 lb | 200 lb |
| --- | --- | --- | --- |
| Basketball | 43 | 58 | 73 |
| Bicycling 10 mph | 33 | 45 | 57 |
| Bicycling 15 mph | 56 | 77 | 98 |
| Carpentry | 38 | 52 | 66 |
| Disco dancing | 26 | 36 | 46 |

| | | | |
|---|---|---|---|
| Square dancing (fast) | 32 | 44 | 56 |
| Eating | 6 | 8 | 10 |
| Golfing (pull cart) | 26 | 36 | 46 |
| Jogging 5 mph | 33 | 45 | 57 |
| Ice-/roller-skating | 25 | 34 | 43 |
| Mowing (power) | 16 | 22 | 28 |
| Racquetball | 66 | 90 | 114 |
| Raking leaves | 22 | 30 | 38 |
| Running 7 mph | 56 | 77 | 98 |
| Running 9 mph | 76 | 103 | 130 |
| Scrubbing floors | 18 | 25 | 32 |
| Shoveling | 33 | 45 | 57 |
| Shoveling snow | 33 | 45 | 57 |
| Skiing | 55 | 75 | 95 |
| Softball | 18 | 25 | 32 |
| Swim 20 yds/min | 26 | 36 | 46 |
| Tennis (doubles) | 21 | 28 | 35 |
| Tennis (singles) | 28 | 38 | 48 |
| Walking 3 mph | 15 | 21 | 27 |
| Waterskiing | 32 | 44 | 56 |

Let's go on now with a totally different kind of question from a woman who was disturbed about the unusual amount of facial hair she had developed. She wanted to know if her diabetes had caused this.

**DR. LOIS:** Once upon a time a teacher of mine in medical school announced that he could always tell a woman with diabetes by whether she had a mustache. I immediately became alarmed, for I always thought that my subtle upper-lip hairs were there because of my Mediterranean background. His statement haunted me, and I then began scrutinizing the upper lip of all my diabetic female patients. My professor was clearly wrong—not all diabetic women have mustaches. But a lot of them do.

Then about five years ago I read an article on the increased prevalence of hirsutism (overgrowth of hair) in women with a long duration of diabetes. The article claimed that prolonged use of insulin is associated with elevations in the male hormone, testosterone, which stimulates facial-hair growth. However, not all faces have numerous potential hair follicles. Therefore, the testosterone would have no effect on hair growth in a fair-skinned Scandinavian woman, whereas a dark-haired lass like me tends to have hair growth.

If the testosterone level is up for any reason, hair will grow. For example, testosterone levels are normally highest at the time of ovulation, and many women note that they need to shave more frequently during this time than any other time of the month.

There is a form of diabetes—overweight Type II— that has markedly elevated insulin levels because of severe insulin resistance. These high levels of insulin thicken the outer coating of the ovary and cause it to turn into a testosterone factory. If these women have the genetic tendency toward dark hair follicles on their faces, they will grow more hair.

The treatment of hairiness includes both decreasing the testosterone level and destroying the hair follicles with electrolysis.

JUNE AND BARBARA: More and more diabetic women are traveling for both business and pleasure, and that of course leads to more and more questions. One frequent-flyer businesswoman wrote to ask if she would have any problem taking her meter and strips through an airport security X-ray machine. We contacted all the meter manufacturers and received the information that none of the meters or strips would be damaged by the X ray. A couple of the manufacturers said that although it isn't necessary, if you wanted to be 100 percent certain of no damage, the meter and strips could be placed in one of the leaded bags used for film. But if it's not necessary, why hassle yourself unduly? Most people don't even use leaded bags for film anymore.

Since pumps are being used more extensively, we thought we'd better check to see if the X ray could mess up their programming, so we checked with Linda Fredrickson, M.A., R.N., C.D.E., of MiniMed, and she said that there is no problem with damaging the pump, although very occasionally it may set off the metal detector alarm. She did caution pump wearers to remember to change the pump clock when passing through time zones.

We think it's always wise to carry along a diabetic ID but especially wise to carry it when you travel to show security guards or customs or anyone who might challenge you for carrying needles or jet injectors or insulin pens or for wearing a pump.

As a jet-setter in your own right, Dr. Lois, winging off to diabetes conferences all over the world, we know you can field all our questions on travel. First off, since most long-distance travel is done on a plane, do you have any tips on dealing with airline food?

DR. LOIS: Sometimes when I have a choice, I fly after dinner. From 8 P.M. onward the airlines do not generally serve food. Although you can request a special "diabetic meal," most airlines make only one generic sick tray. This is an all-purpose meal for everyone with some kind of ailment, be it peptic-ulcer disease, high blood pressure, kidney disease, or diabetes. Consequently, it is bland, saltless, sugarless, and tasteless. I would much rather pick and choose from a normal tray. If the meal is composed of too many forbidden foods, my carry-on has a supply of supplements.

JUNE AND BARBARA: If you travel with a cooperative friend and eat the regular meal there's often a choice of entrees. You and your friend can each order a different one and then you can select the meal—or parts of each meal—that is best for your diet.

After the vagaries of in-flight meals are taken care of, the prime problem every traveling diabetic woman has to deal with is jet lag. Even after all these years of travel, June still has trouble keeping her blood sugars normal after a flight through time zones. Maybe you could first enlighten us on what jet lag is, aside from making a traveler starkly awake when she should be sleeping and totally groggy when she should be awake.

DR. LOIS: The hypothalamus (seat of the wake-sleep cycle) is programmed by light and darkness. When we change the light/dark cycle by greater than an hour, there needs to be a resetting of the hypothalamus to accommodate to these shifts. When a person flies from California to New York, the three-hour change is enough to disrupt the body's internal clock.

Our insulin requirement varies throughout the day, with greater needs during the early-morning waking hours (4 A.M. to 10 A.M.) and lesser needs during deep sleep (12 midnight to 4 A.M.). If our wristwatch time is shifted three hours but our hypothalamus does not adjust to that fact for a period of time (usually one day for every hour of time-zone change)—then timing of insulin becomes a challenge. If our Californian goes all the way to Germany, there is a nine-hour time change, and as a result everything may be topsy-turvy for up to nine days. The best way to handle travel through different time zones is to make an appointment with your physician to talk about insulin adjustments. Bring the flight times and time-zone changes and know the number of meals served on the airplane. Please do not just call your doctor and ask advice over the phone. You deserve a carefully thought-out plan of action.

JUNE AND BARBARA: Alas, what you deserve and what you get are often two different things these days. We hear from more and more people who are in HMOs that they have a gatekeeper who acts more like a hockey goalie blocking them from getting to an endocrinologist unless they are in dire straits. This gatekeeper doesn't have the time or, frankly, the expertise to advise on travel insulin adjustments. Could you give people in that situation some guidelines?

DR. LOIS: I generally tell patients to take their usual dose of Regular (short-acting) before the dinner on a flight to Europe and then skip the long-acting insulin (which is usually NPH) because the time change is nine hours from L.A. or six hours from New York, and these hours are lost. When the flight attendant wakes the passengers for "breakfast," take the daytime long- and short-acting insulin and immediately reset your watch and assume the European time. Then you should measure your blood sugars every two to three hours for at least a week to carefully adjust the insulin up or down as needed.

JUNE AND BARBARA: June always has a much more difficult time when she goes from west to east than from east to west, even though the flights usually take longer when you're flying west because of the headwinds.

DR. LOIS: Almost everyone finds it easier to adjust to east-to-west time-zone changes. A longer day with more sunlight helps the hypothalamus to adjust faster. In this east-to-west situation you merely add a dose of Regular for the four meals eaten: breakfast in Europe, lunch and dinner on the plane, and another dinner at home. Then take the long-acting insulin on the home time as usual. Here again, increasing the blood-sugar checking for a week allows the fine-tuning to take place.

JUNE AND BARBARA: We've been hearing from traveling friends about the benefits of taking synthetic melatonin (available at health-food stores) at night to help you sleep and thereby to alleviate the effects of jet lag. The *British Medical Journal* reported on a study that seemed to confirm that it works. What is this melatonin and what does it do?

DR. LOIS: Melatonin is a human hormone derivative of the amino acid tryptophane. At night the pineal gland releases melatonin, which makes you sleepy. During the day the light suppresses the release of melatonin, so you feel awake. It is thought that melatonin helps adjust the hypothalamus through the wake/sleep cycle.

JUNE AND BARBARA: The only thing that bothers us about melatonin is that they're starting to make a lot of outlandish claims about other benefits from it such as protecting against aging, heart disease, Parkinson's, Alzheimer's, retarding the growth of certain tumors, and increasing your sexual prowess. Sounds kind of like the claims made in the past for vitamin C and vitamin E and other supplements that had their periods of faddish favor. The only side effect mentioned in writeups of melatonin is that in some women it acts as a mild contraceptive. (Maybe that's because it puts you to sleep at night.) At any rate, do you know of any reason why a diabetic—or anyone else, for that matter—should not use melatonin to speed recovery from jet lag.

**DR. LOIS:** No, the research seems to show that it is safe and useful. I recommend the standard dose of 5 to 10 mg of melatonin taken thirty to ninety minutes before bedtime for as many nights as the jet-lag feelings persist.

**JUNE AND BARBARA:** As a bon voyage present, we think some of the last words of caution for diabetic travelers from your book *The Diabetes Self-Care Method* bear repeating here. Can you summarize them briefly?

**DR. LOIS:** I always recommend carrying enough pocket food to treat low blood sugar. Since your internal clock is changing slowly to adjust to the abrupt time change, your insulin may act more strongly than it usually does, so you need to have food along at all times. This is especially true in a foreign place. Trying to speak another language and make a food purchase with foreign money is a tough-enough task, let alone during an insulin reaction.

The exercise level of a traveler is also unpredictable. The travel may involve virtually no exercise (as in the case of traveling or sightseeing by car, train, bus, or plane) or all exercise (as in the case of a biking or walking tour). The pocket food comes in handy for the days when exercise turns out to be more than you anticipated when you took your morning dose of insulin. It would also be wise to carry a syringe with Regular in it or an insulin pen in order to take extra insulin on days with little exercise—or in case the tour bus stops in front of the best pastry shop in all of Europe.

JUNE AND BARBARA: Another problem that some diabetic working women have to deal with is shift work. Despite all the Americans with Disabilities Act claims to the contrary, when your diabetes schedule conflicts with your work schedule, employers often aren't willing to make adjustments for you. We've received many questions about shift work and other work schedule/medication problems. One woman on oral medication was told by her doctor to take her pills *exactly* twelve hours apart and her job schedule made this hard to do, because she was being required to do a lot of overtime. Is it that crucial that she take her pills *exactly* twelve hours apart? How much leeway is possible?

DR. LOIS: Some oral medications are very short acting and serve to improve the blood-sugar response to food (glipizide, Glynase, a pulvarized glyburide). Other oral agents are longer acting and serve to help the between-meal blood sugars (glyburide). However, the pills should be taken to achieve the best possible control. Sometimes I prescribe the glyburide to be taken before bedtime to conquer tomorrow's morning blood glucose (fasting). I use it as though it were NPH insulin at bedtime. Thus, the every-twelve-hour schedule does not make sense if the timing does not match the lifestyle and the resultant blood sugars. Everything depends on the kind of oral agents you're taking and your particular work-schedule problems.

JUNE AND BARBARA: How about insulin takers? How do they handle changing schedules and different sleeping patterns on weekends. One doctor said this was such a difficult situation that a pump would be the only solution. He compared it to trying to use a little Miata sports car on terrain where a four-wheel drive, off-road vehicle was required. Not everyone can afford a pump and not all insurance plans will pay for one. Have you a less-expensive solution?

DR. LOIS: Shift working for an insulin-taking person requires two completely different doses of insulin: one for daytime work schedules and one for nighttime workdays. The person's blood-sugar records need to be kept for five days of the daytime schedule and five days of the nighttime schedule. When visiting your prescribing physician, you should lay out the following information:

### 1. Five days of daytime schedule:
Meals, times, exercise, insulin doses, high stress times, and 8 blood sugars a day—before each meal, one hour after each meal, at bedtime and at 3 A.M.

### 2. Five days of nighttime schedule:
Meals, times, exercise, insulin doses, high stress times, and 8 blood sugars—before each meal, one hour after each meal, when you go to sleep, when you wake up and another halfway in between sleep and wakeup.

Armed with this much information, a physician can devise two different insulin plans. The doses of Regular insulin should be timed before the meals, which are at different times on days than nights. The basal needs can be covered using two doses of an intermediate insulin or a long-acting insulin such as ultralente.

JUNE AND BARBARA: From this it's easy to see how important it is to adjust your insulin to your life and activities, but not all women receive the necessary guidance to do make these adjustments. A nurse working in a rest home said the elderly staff doctor—we'll call him Dr. Coot—was known for his standard insulin dosage—twenty units of NPH—for everyone who had diabetes. When a patient in the rest home was diagnosed diabetic, the nurses sighed and said, "She'll just be put on the standard 'Coot shot,'" and she always was.

On this same subject, a thirty-nine-year-old woman wrote us that after reading the first edition of *The Diabetic Woman* she realized she was "in big danger." She had been a Type I diabetic for thirty-five years and because she had only had what she called "doctors from hell," she had been on the same fifteen units of Regular insulin and thirty units of NPH every A.M. without ever changing the dosage for fifteen years. She didn't regularly check her blood sugar, but when she did "it tended to run high." She realized for the first time that she was "a walking time bomb," and she wanted help and suggestions from you. There must be other "time bombs" out there, too, who need rescuing from the "standard dose jungle."

DR. LOIS: When the pancreas does not secrete insulin, then we must be smart enough to take our insulin doses to match our weight, state of stress, our menstrual cycle, our exercise, and the food we eat. One dose of insulin cannot fit every day, and thus we must learn to adjust the insulin to match our lifestyles. It is totally impossible to adjust our lifestyles to fit someone's standard dose of insulin.

To begin to conquer your blood sugars, you need intensive education about your own metabolism and about the pharmacology of insulin (timing, onset, duration, absorption characteristics, etc.). In order to learn how to self-manage your blood sugars, you need to perform blood sugars at crucial time points. Devising an insulin system for you requires that you perform eight blood-glucose levels a day (before and one hour after each meal, and at bedtime and at 3 A.M.). These blood sugars will guide a health-care team to help you conquer your sugars. To find a diabetes team certified by the American Diabetes Association, call your local ADA (the number is in the white pages of the phone book).

JUNE AND BARBARA: Many of these walking-time-bomb women are in HMOs with gatekeepers who won't let them go to an endocrinologist and who have no diabetes care team to help make these vitally necessary adjustments. The only solution we can think of for this is to make the personal investment of going to an endocrinologist or a hospital program with a diabetes-care team to get yourself on track and take the information back to the HMO primary-care physician to work with. But this is an expensive solution that is flat-out impossible for many women. Do you have any suggestions as to how they can handle it?

DR. LOIS: Many endocrinologists are also primary-care providers in order to make ends meet. After all, they must first be internists before they become endocrinologists. A quick cross-reference of the names in the primary-care list and the endocrinology list may show that indeed there are endocrinologists working as primary-care physicians and you could request one of those. If there are none, nephrologists may also exist in the primary-care lists. Kidney doctors believe tight control prevents kidney problems, so one of them would make a very good diabetes doctor. It's well worth your time to do this detective work at your HMO.

JUNE AND BARBARA: Sometimes no matter how hard you try, you ultimately can't get to a physician at the HMO who can effectively treat your diabetes. Sometimes, in fact, the HMO won't even allow you the equipment and supplies you need for tight control, for example enough strips for the testing you must do or even a pump if all else fails. A diabetes specialist we were talking to at the ADA Conference when the DCCT results revealed that tight control prevents complications, said that this means diabetics now have legal grounds to force HMOs to give them proper treatment or they can sue for damages if the treatment has been refused and complications result. We don't like to recommend suing. There's already too much of that in our society. (We believe in the old saying that "litigation is a machine in which you enter as a pig and emerge as sausage.") Besides, it doesn't seem like the best solution to get complications and sue for damages. Do you have any alternatives?

DR. LOIS: There is hope for the future, and it's not too far away. Soon—maybe by the time you read this—"standard care" practice will incorporate the principles of tight control for diabetes. We can thank the DCCT for that. A little patience will reward those who wait by giving them all the tools and techniques for good diabetes control, compliments of a universal health-care policy.

JUNE AND BARBARA: Diabetic women often report that they keep having mood swings. Is this due to hypoglycemia or hyperglycemia?

DR. LOIS: Both! Hypoglycemia may be subtle and can present itself as anger or depression. Hyperglycemia may show itself as anxiety, irritability, and/or unstable emotions. Improved glucose control improves mood, and improved mood improves glucose control.

JUNE AND BARBARA: Speaking of hypoglycemia, we often get questions about it, not as a condition occurring in insulin-dependent diabetes (or even with the oral hypoglycemic pills) but as a separate disease in the nondiabetic population. People who have it—or think they have it—probably come to us for information because they have nowhere else to turn. There are no authoritative and comprehensive books on the subject, and many doctors consider it a nondisease or even a cult. We usually suggest to them that they can check themselves in the same way people with diabetes do by taking their blood sugar when they feel the symptoms of irritability and shakiness.

Another reason they seek us out is that they've heard that hypoglycemia is sometimes a precursor of diabetes. Could you shed some light on all this murkiness?

DR. LOIS: Many of these nondiabetic people probably suffer from a normal condition called "reactive hypoglycemia." It is caused by eating a pure carbohydrate meal like a breakfast of toast and juice. Three or four hours later they feel irritable and shaky, because their blood sugar has dropped to around 40 mg/dl. It is estimated that 40 percent of all lean persons go down to 40 mg/dl if they don't eat for four hours after a pure-carbohydrate meal. Therefore, reactive hypoglycemia is a normal response, but that doesn't make it any less uncomfortable to experience. It can be alleviated by eating mixed meals with adequate fat and protein.

As for hypoglycemia being a precursor of diabetes, people who have high blood sugar one hour after a meal (with *high* being defined as over 200 mg/dl) and who then "crash" from 200 down to 40 do have a higher risk of diabetes, perhaps double the risk of people in the general population.

JUNE AND BARBARA: In days gone by, a woman's role was defined as that of *Kinder, Kirche, Küche*—children, church, and cooking. While the modern woman certainly isn't confined to these three, we have noticed in the questions we receive that many women still seem to be the defenders of the faith and tend to worry more than men about possible conflicts between their religion and their diabetes care.

For example, a diabetes nurse educator got in touch with us because she was concerned about a patient who was an insulin-taking diabetic woman. The patient was a member of the Christian Science church and was planning to take a trip with friends who were members of the same church. Her friends didn't know that this woman was a diabetic person, and she didn't plan to tell them because she was ashamed of taking insulin, feeling it showed a lack of faith. The nurse was worried that if the woman had a reaction, no one would know what was going on and they wouldn't know how to help her.

We wrote to the board of directors of the First Church of Christ, Scientist in Boston and received a thoughtful response from the manager of the committees on publication. It is such a lucid and caring letter that we recommend that anyone who may be wrestling with such a decision read it in its entirety (if you write to us at Prana Publications 5623 Matilija Ave., Van Nuys, CA 91401, we'll be glad to send you a copy). We would like to include this brief excerpt here:

As for guilt feelings, I don't think these ordinarily would (or should) be a problem for a Christian Scientist who has decided to seek medical help. The teachings of Christian Science simply do not point a condemning finger at such individuals, much less equate sickness simplistically with "lack of faith." Nor does the church encourage the view that those who use medicine are somehow committing a sin. A Christian Scientist who turns to a doctor in [a] difficult circumstance would be less apt to dwell on feelings of failure than to resolve all the more to work and pray for the spiritual understanding and closeness to God that is, we believe, the ultimate source for freedom and healing. This would be as true in the case of someone electing to use insulin for an indefinite period as it would be in any other situation.

In your practice, have you ever come across problems of religion or philosophy in conflict with diabetes control—for example, a person who wanted to fast for religious reasons?

DR. LOIS: Yes, this has happened. Fortunately, the Jewish law exempts pregnant and nursing women from fasting. So far, most of my patients' fasting has not been a problem, but we have had to make some very clever maneuvers with insulin to allow for Jewish ritualistic foods, such as matzo (a very high-carbohydrate, unleavened bread), Manischewitz wine (which is sweeter than grape juice), and honey and apples, which are a customary part of welcoming the New Year.

A greater challenge is the Indian diet, which is devoid of meat and is 70 percent carbohydrate. All these special situations require changes in insulin, but so far we seem to have found ways to keep the religion *and* to keep the sugar controlled.

JUNE AND BARBARA: On the other hand, following the tenets of certain religions can be a positive factor in diabetes. The *American Journal of Public Health* proposed the thesis that a vegetarian diet reduces the risk of developing diabetes. Based on a twenty-one-year study of a population of 25,698 white adult Seventh-Day Adventists (most of whom follow a vegetarian diet), diabetes was found to be the underlying cause of death in the men of this faith at half the rate that diabetes causes death in all U.S. white males.

While we're on this subject, June demands equal time for Buddhism, which is as much a philosophy as a religion. We find that diabetics and those who work with diabetics are well advised to strive for the four Buddhist virtues: joy, friendliness, compassion, and equanimity. This last word has a richness of meaning. The dictionary defines it as "emotional or mental stability or composure, especially under tension or strain; calmness, equilibrium." Think what developing these virtues would do for controlling your diabetes and enhancing your life!

And here's a Buddhist thought that could apply equally well to diabetes and to any other adversity you may be called upon to face: Bless your enemy, for he enables you to grow.

# 2 ❧ *A*ges and Stages

THEY ORDER THE MATTER OF AGES AND STAGES BETTER IN France than in the United States. Take, for example, the Miss/Mrs. controversy that we've tried—for the most part unsuccessfully—to resolve with the hybrid Ms. In France there's no problem. You're Mademoiselle until you marry or reach that indeterminate *un certain âge*, at which time you automatically become Madame.

Then there's the nomenclatural wrestling that we do in this country when referring to people who are, shall we say, mature. We've tried "senior citizen" (ugh!) and "the elderly," both of which conjure up visions of decrepitude, and we've also tried such euphemisms as "the golden years." In France, there is no problem—this stage of life is called simply and straightforwardly *le troisième âge* (the third age).

In keeping with this, and following an *Alice in Wonderland* admonition, "Speak in French, remember who you are," we're going to divide the woman diabetic's ages and stages into *le premier âge, le deuxième âge*, and *le troisième âge*. In the first of these we'll discuss childhood and puberty to the extent that as far as diabetes is concerned, these ages differ for girls and young women in comparison to those of the masculine persuasion. Because we did not receive many questions from children, adolescents, or their parents, and neither June nor Lois nor Barbara has a diabetic child, in this section we will deal primarily with Type I diabetes in general. It's this type that generally appears during the first third of life.

In *le deuxième âge*, we'll cover the events that usually occur in this period: career choices, marriage, and pregnancy.

In *le* good old *troisième âge*, we'll not only go into the significant physiological and psychological aspects of menopause but we'll also explore Type II diabetes, both generally and specifically, because the majority of cases of this type of diabetes come to light during this period of life.

And so, *Mademoiselles* and *Mesdames*, let's get to it, or, in other words, *allons-y*.

## Le Premier Age

Gail Sheehy, writing in her book *The Spirit of Survival*, says:

> Sudden or disorienting change introduced into the family or social and political environment of a child does not necessarily leave permanent scars on the temperament. Quite the contrary. Adversity is part of life, and learning to master adversity is one of the basic ways of gaining self-confidence and self-esteem. Disorders of behavior that may develop while a child or adolescent is in the midst of a crisis often subside or disappear once a consistency of environ-

ment and relationships is reestablished. And the experience of knowing one has survived can offer a psychological shield against future disasters in adult life.

We were discussing this with Dr. Jovanovic, and she echoed Gail Sheehy's sentiment. "I truly believe," she said, "that behind every great woman is a child who has had to suffer in one way or another."

We all agree, however, that there's no point in just suffering for suffering's sake. Therefore, in this section we'll try to present information that will keep suffering at a minimum for the diabetic girl and Type I woman and develop coping skills that will minimize diabetes problems.

We cannot here go into every aspect of being or raising a diabetic child. That would fill an entire book on its own. Please refer to the Parents and Children section in Recommended Reading, where you'll find books for mothers and fathers and for young diabetic readers.

JUNE AND BARBARA: We've heard some mothers of diabetic babies and very small children say that they prefer to do urine tests because they can't bear to stick the little fingers. Do you think that it's okay to substitute urine tests in this case?

DR. LOIS: No. The smaller the child, the more important it is to know what the blood sugar is immediately. Hypoglycemia presents itself in peculiar ways in infants, especially ones who do not talk yet.

JUNE AND BARBARA: Given the smallness of their fingers, how often do you think children this little should have blood sugars taken?

DR. LOIS: Even if their fingers are small, they do have ten of them—and ten toes as well—so there are sufficient places from which to take the blood samples. I feel that at least three times a day is not too often for infants and small children to have blood-sugar tests.

JUNE AND BARBARA: Do you believe that it's a good idea for diabetic girls and teenagers to attend special diabetes camps?

DR. LOIS: Yes, yes, a thousand times yes! I don't know how many times I have had young women tell me that they felt terribly alone as adolescents. Diabetes embarrassed them so they hid it; rather than sleeping over at a girlfriend's house and risk being found out, they chose to be alone.

The camp experience is wonderful. The campers, and even most of the counselors, have diabetes. The child immediately feels part of the majority. Insulin therapy, diet, and the camp experience are all molded into one. Once a camper learns how to adjust the diet and insulin to compensate for the track meet, the swimming competition, the campout, and the hike, then she's ready for a camp that does not specialize in diabetes.

Simply asking a regular camp to "watch out" for a diabetic child is inviting the child to a summer of chance—the chance that nothing bad will happen. There are more than thirty camps in America for diabetic children. Surely one would fit any child's special interests and still be a place where diabetes skills can be reinforced. Call your local American Diabetes Association for information on summer camps.

JUNE AND BARBARA: We especially agree with how important it is for the diabetic child to feel part of the majority for a change. We think that's good for diabetics of all ages.

Barbara, a *non*diabetic and the co-author of so many diabetes books, can feel a little awkward and out of place at get-togethers for diabetics. Whenever she is talking with people at such gatherings and they ask with a hopeful smile, "Are *you* a diabetic?" she always looks down in embarrassment, scuffs her toe against the carpet, and has to admit, "Well, no, actually I'm not." But she adds, quickly, "I try to live as if I am one, though!" She says that in these situations she feels like the outcast member of a certain tribe in South America in which almost everyone has a goiter because of a lack of iodine, a genetic trait, or both. When a child, through some quirk of nature, does not develop a goiter, his little friends taunt him, saying things like "Nyah, nyah, bottleneck."

DR. LOIS: It's good for everybody to have these reverse experiences from time to time in order to see how the other half feels.

JUNE AND BARBARA: When a young girl begins to menstruate, does this affect her diabetes in any way?

DR. LOIS: With the beginning of menstruation or puberty, control of blood sugars usually deteriorates—as reflected by rising glycosylated hemoglobin levels—even though the doctors tend to increase insulin doses. In fact, unstable diabetes is a common problem in young patients with Type I diabetes, particularly during adolescence.

This deterioration of control is usually blamed on the psychosocial upheavals in an adolescent's life or on cheating on the diet. However, a study by Dr. Stephanie Amiel published in the *New England Journal of Medicine* clearly showed that it is the high levels of maturation hormones that cause the diabetes to be out of control if the insulin dose is not doubled.

Thus, puberty is a time when the insulin dose needs to be adjusted upward. The largest dose of insulin tends to be the overnight insulin dose, because the highest secretion of growth hormone and the sex hormones is at the point of deepest sleeping. Since the growth hormone and the sex hormones are anti-insulin in action, the insulin dose of necessity needs to be adjusted upward.

One mystery is why diabetic complications never occur before puberty, no matter how many years the diabetes has existed. It is almost as though the complications time clock doesn't start ticking off the years until after the onset of menstruation. It is hoped that tight control may stop this clock.

JUNE AND BARBARA: We've had a lot of questions from women who find that their blood sugar goes up unexpectedly just before the onset of their menstrual period. (Actually, it isn't unexpected, since it happens every month!) Is this a common occurrence?

DR. LOIS: Yes. It's quite usual for blood sugars to go up markedly between two and five days before the menstrual period.

JUNE AND BARBARA: Why is this?

DR. LOIS: Throughout the course of the menstrual cycle, levels of various hormones in a woman's body change drastically. Let me review for you the normal menstrual cycle to make clear what happens and when.

The normal cycle has two phases. The first, or follicular, phase has its onset on day one, coincident with the onset of menses. During this first phase, the female hormones—specifically, estrogen and progesterone—are at their lowest levels. These two hormones exert an action against insulin. When their levels are low, insulin seems stronger. In other words, less insulin is required to keep the blood sugar normal, even if food intake is not altered.

By day fourteen, or midway through the cycle, the pituitary releases another hormone, luteinizing hormone (LH), which causes an egg (ovum) to be released from the ovary. This starts the second, or luteal, phase of the cycle. The egg then travels down a tube (the fallopian tube) to the womb (uterus).

Meanwhile, the egg's old wrappings in the ovary turn into a hormone factory (corpus luteum) and secrete large quantities of estrogen and progesterone to prepare the uterine lining (endometrium) for the nestling-in of the ovum if the ovum perchance meets its counterpart, the sperm, swimming up the tube. In this chance encounter, if the ovum and sperm are united (conception), they arrive as one unit (the trophoblast) to take up housekeeping in the warm, boggy, prepared endometrium.

If the ovum is not fertilized, it will not nestle into the endometrium but will merely wash out of the vagina. The corpus luteum, which produced the estrogen and progesterone to prepare the endometrium, knows that it is not needed because conception did not occur. If conception occurs, another hormone produced by the trophoblast signals the corpus luteum to produce estrogen and progesterone. This hormone, human chorionic gonadotropin (HCG), is the hormone that turns pregnancy tests positive. Without this hormone signal to the corpus luteum, the production of estrogen and progesterone ceases. The lack of these two hormones to nourish the endometrium causes the endometrium to shed, a phenomenon we call menses.

Since estrogen and progesterone counteract insulin, the action of insulin is weaker during the luteal phase. Since estrogen and progesterone are the highest during the last week of the cycle, this week requires the most insulin. In other words, it takes more insulin to keep the blood sugar normal even where there is no change in food intake.

JUNE AND BARBARA: How does a woman go about adjusting her insulin to accommodate all of this?

DR. LOIS: Once she begins to ovulate, a woman's hormone pattern should be fairly consistent and predictable, even though the hormone levels may vary slightly from month to month. By learning from one month's insulin requirement, you can make an informed decision about how much insulin to take next month. The first step is to discover when these hormone surges occur. Since you may not feel any different, the only sure way to tell is to watch the calendar and test your blood as soon as you get up every morning. You want to know the *fasting* blood-glucose level, so you should monitor your blood sugar before you eat breakfast.

When you know that this rise is occurring, you can slowly increase your insulin dosage, particularly in the overnight insulins, which are designed to have you in the normal range of blood sugar when you wake up. Since estrogen and progesterone are working against insulin throughout this five-day period, you need to have slightly more insulin circulating in your blood the entire time. This means that you require slightly more long-acting insulin (NPH, lente, or ultralente insulin), or, if you're using the insulin pump, more "basal" flow of regular insulin.

The insulin dosage should be raised *very gradually* (by perhaps 3 percent a day over a five-day period). This may not be enough to get your blood-sugar level back to normal the first month, but at least you'll know where to start your dosage when the next month rolls around. As soon as you see the first stain of blood, immediately drop the insulin dose back to the original starting dosage, because the estrogen and progesterone levels have already dropped back to their normal baseline levels. It's important to decrease the insulin dosage at this time so that you don't have an episode of low blood sugar in the middle of the night. As always, you should consult your own physician before changing your insulin dosage.

JUNE AND BARBARA: We hear a lot about premenstrual syndrome (PMS) these days. Could you define it and describe how it might particularly affect diabetic women?

DR. LOIS: Premenstrual syndrome is a term that is used very loosely. Many women have some symptoms—bloating or increased water retention, menstrual cramps, acne, irritability, and depression—that are caused by high levels of progesterone in the blood. However, the term *premenstrual syndrome* applies only if these symptoms are incapacitating and interfere with work or home life.

If you have these symptoms and feel overwhelmed by them, your physician can give you a medication that can help to alleviate them after simple dietary changes have been made, such as avoiding salty foods, caffeine, and chocolate. Antiprostaglandin agents are the best, for prostaglandin has been implicated as the major villain.

Motrin is a very strong antiprostaglandin that I recommend to my patients. It's best to discuss these symptoms in conjunction with your premenstrual insulin requirements during the same visit to your physician.

You may also find that you can ease some of your moody feelings by keeping your blood sugar in good control. There has been scientific evidence to suggest that high blood sugar can contribute to depression, making premenstrual moodiness even worse. The anxiety you feel can raise your blood sugar even higher, so do try to keep your blood sugar in good control, even through these turbulent periods—because we all know those times are tough enough already!

Remember the credo "Know thyself." This is good advice in general, but it is particularly relevant to the woman with diabetes. By learning all you can about your own monthly cycle, you can gradually achieve and maintain that wholesome balance that keeps you feeling good.

JUNE AND BARBARA: We've had frequent pleas for help from women who experience extreme, virtually uncontrollable food cravings just before the onset of their periods. One arrived after the publication of *Diabetes Type II and What to Do* on which we collaborated with Virginia Valentine, R.N., M.S., C.D.E., who is a diabetes educator and a Type II diabetic, herself. We forwarded that letter to Virginia and this was her response:

> You are getting cravings before your period because of hormone changes that occur during that time of the month. Of course, knowing this doesn't make the cravings go away. How to manage these cravings? Give in! People who try to be restrictive with their diets often end up binging later. Instead of focusing on what you can't have, take a look at some goodies you *can* have and plan them into your diet.

Have some of the fruited fat-free yogurts on hand (the ones with Nutrasweet that have only 90 to 100 calories) for a filling, yet healthy and sweet snack. Wax Orchards makes a fudge sauce (Fudge Sweet) that is *to die for*. This stuff is amazing, it tastes like a truly sinful thick fudge sauce but it has only 16 calories per teaspoon and is fat free! You can create some awesome desserts with it, put it on diet ice cream, dip strawberries in it, or drizzle it over strawberries on top of angel food cake. For a quick chocolate fix, spread some on a vanilla wafer and put another wafer on top, there you have it: a reverse Oreo cookie! Make up some sugar-free pudding and then put lite Cool Whip on top. A patient told me the other day that they now have lite Cool Whip in chocolate flavor. You could mix that with some sugar-free chocolate pudding and create a pretty awesome chocolate mousse. As you can see, you have really hit on one of my favorite topics! Be creative, plan ahead, and when you focus on what you can have, you can avoid the deprivation mode that is so destructive to diets and emotional well-being.

Debra Waterhouse, in her book *Why Women Need Chocolate*, echoes Virginia's sentiment of "give in to your cravings." In fact she says that your cravings are an indication of what your body needs, going so far as to say, "Food cravings are not a problem to be treated, but a blessing to be encouraged." She explains that women are more likely to crave chocolate, crackers, ice cream, and fruit while men are more likely to crave meat, eggs, hot dogs, pizza, and seafood. However, she has no specific information on food cravings that women with diabetes have—nor any suggestions like Virginia's on how they can handle these cravings without wrecking their blood sugar. Do diabetic women have the same ones as nondiabetic women, or do they have different ones or both of the above?

**DR. LOIS:** Diabetic women are normal, and so they have normal cravings. The increase in progesterone during the premenstrual period drives these cravings. "Giving in" releases the tension also associated with progesterone elevations.

**JUNE AND BARBARA:** Do these food cravings generally diminish after menopause?

**DR. LOIS:** Yes, however diabetic women should not be denied their hormones! The doses of progesterone necessary to keep us healthy may reinitiate these cravings, but many times the progesterone needed is less than the levels required to elicit these cravings. Thus, clever adjustment of hormones may be necessary.

**JUNE AND BARBARA:** While on the subject of menstruation, we wrote in our first book, *Alice in Womanland*, about the pamphlets and women's magazine articles that "tell the newly pubertized girl who lies clutching a heating pad to her cramped innards, 'But, my dear, don't call it the *curse*. It's part of the *joy* of being a woman. It's a blessing and you should be happy to experience it, and, yes, *proud*.'" This struck us as so ludicrous that we took to referring to our monthly periods ironically as "the joy" or, with the delicacy of the French language, *"la joie."* At any rate, whether you regard cramps as pain or rapture, what causes them and how can they be avoided or gotten rid of?

**DR. LOIS:** The chief cause of cramps is prostaglandins, which make the uterus contract. Any antiprostaglandin will work to prevent cramps, but high doses are needed, and many of these drugs have severe side effects at higher doses. Motrin (ibuprofen), which I mentioned before, has few side effects. Ordinary aspirin will work, too, but many times high dosages of aspirin are irritating to the stomach.

**JUNE AND BARBARA:** Is there anything wrong with over-the-counter drugs like Midol?

**DR. LOIS:** No, there's nothing wrong with them if they work. But for those who suffer from severe cramps my advice is to build up blood levels with drugs five days before the period is due. For example, take 400 mg of ibuprofen four times a day, at breakfast, lunch, dinner, and bedtime. This acts to contract the prostaglandins as they pour into the bloodstream *before* the cramps occur. It's much harder to stop cramps once they start.

**JUNE AND BARBARA:** Are diabetic women more susceptible to cramps than nondiabetic women?

**DR. LOIS:** No. Poor diabetic control may prevent ovulation, and lack of ovulation is a reason for missed or scanty periods. But control doesn't seem to impact on the degree of pain of menstrual cramps.

Cramps are the normal pain response to a uterus clamping down to get rid of the old blood and tissue. Why the uterine muscle hurts so much when it contracts nobody knows. The Bible claims that labor pains are our punishment for partaking of the golden apple—but it doesn't seem fair that we feel this pain every month!

**JUNE AND BARBARA:** Everything we've discussed so far makes it sound as if all girls and women diagnosed in *le première âge* are Type I's. Is this always the case?

DR. LOIS: No, while it is almost always the case, there is a type of diabetes called MODY. This stands for "Maturity Onset Diabetes of Youth." It literally means that "adult onset" diabetes happens to children and young women. There is a very strong family history, and usually one parent and all the kids have it. It is also associated with acceleration of complications if the diabetes is not under good control. MODY can either be the lean, Type II insulin-sensitive type diabetes or the insulin-resistant classic obesity-associated diabetes. For the lean Type II, insulin is probably the treatment of choice. For the insulin resistant, diet and exercise are the mainstays of therapy.

JUNE AND BARBARA: As you might imagine, many young—and not quite so young—women have written us with questions about sex. Most of these questions can be boiled down to this: How does diabetes affect one's sex life?

DR. LOIS: Sex is so simple to spell, yet so difficult to talk about. Perhaps it is our upbringing that pushes sex into the whispers of our conversations; perhaps it is our own insecurity that we are not good enough, not worthy enough, or not fortunate enough. But sex should be quite natural—after all, it is a bodily function. Diabetic women have the same wonder about sex as nondiabetic women. The main difference is that if any small problem arises, many women have hidden fears that it is something about having diabetes that creates the problem.

There are some situations that do impact on sex when a woman has diabetes. One example in particular comes to mind. If a woman thoroughly enjoys the sexual encounter, the sheer exercise of the experience may result in a severe hypoglycemic episode. Thus, a woman needs to be prepared. She should adjust her insulin downward in anticipation of the evening, or, if the event happens on the spur of the moment, she should compensate by eating something afterward.

*Libido* is the word that describes our lust for sex. Psychological as well as hormonal factors control our libido. If a woman is sick, she certainly has no interest in sex. Likewise, if she is suffering from a severe vaginal infection, she would avoid a sexual encounter because of the fear of pain. High blood-glucose levels tend to be associated with increased problems with vaginitis, and it is therefore not surprising that so many diabetic women do not enjoy sex.

In addition, if the diabetes is out of control to a degree sufficient to cause delayed or missed periods, the normal cycling of hormones that increase libido doesn't occur. There are some diabetic women, on the other hand, who experience an *increase* in libido. These women have a syndrome of diabetes and polycystic ovarian disease that elevates the male hormone testosterone in their blood. Testosterone is the strongest libido-producing hormone.

Libido is also intimately associated with mood. If a woman is depressed, she cannot be easily seduced. In addition, if she does not feel sexy, she is not in the mood for sex. Unfortunately, being overweight is associated with Type II diabetes and also with not feeling sexy. It is true, too, that chronic hyperglycemia is associated with depression, and that's another reason why women with diabetes may not be interested in sex.

The best way to be sexy and enjoy sex, therefore, is to be happy, healthy, fit, and in good control of your blood-glucose levels.

JUNE AND BARBARA: One complaint we've heard is that women are often neglected in studies of sex and diabetes, most of which are concerned with impotence in males.

DR. LOIS: It's true that men have gotten most of the attention, and there are several reasons for this. For one thing, women haven't complained loudly enough in the past. Perhaps the women's movement has taught us to be more assertive now. For another, when a man has no libido he cannot perform, for he will not be able to have an erection. When a woman has decreased libido, while it is true that she will not have adequate lubrication, she can still perform by using a bit of jelly. Finally, the first researchers in this field were men, and thus their interest was primarily in men. We women researchers have been guilty of investigating only female problems, too.

Now that women with diabetes have brought up this issue, a major laboratory at Columbia University has performed elegant studies to document a physiological etiology of decreased libido in certain women with diabetes.

Along with the information I gave you in the previous question, I can add that Dr. Judith Lorber, in her studies at Columbia, found that loss of libido can be caused by the following:

> **Out-of-control diabetes.** Hyperglycemia can potentiate depression and a sense of being hopeless and helpless. Such feelings do not make one feel sexy. In addition, these blood-glucose levels take their toll on energy and vitality and can actually be a form of chronic illness, not to mention causing an increased susceptibility to infections.
> **Vaginal infections, specifically, moniliasis or can-**

**didiasis.** These infections cause a terrible itching and increased pain on intercourse. The fear of pain can be a great turnoff to sex.

**Neuropathy.** Dr. Lorber has documented a form of diabetic neuropathy that affects the nerves to the genital area. This condition can prevent adequate lubrication as well as orgasmic climax. It is the same condition present in the male diabetic person who has impotence on an autonomic neuropathic basis.

JUNE AND BARBARA: Since the one thing a diabetic woman shouldn't have is an unplanned pregnancy before she has achieved the good blood-sugar control that assures a healthy baby, it stands to reason that she is going to have to practice some form of birth control. Could you give us a rundown of the various methods and recommend the ones that are best for diabetic women?

DR. LOIS: To review the latest birth-control options we'll start with the oral contraceptives (the "pill"), because they are 99 percent effective when used correctly. The pill is a combination of female hormones. Although called "oral" contraceptives, they actually come in other dosage forms. Two of these are Depo Provera, administered by injection and active up to three months and Norplant, which consists of device that is implanted just beneath the skin of the upper arm. Its contraceptive effects last for up to five years. All of these forms are available by prescription only.

Oral contraceptives may not be for you if you have a medical history of heart disease, stroke, high blood pressure, or blood vessel problems (such as phlebitis). Your health risks are increased if you're a smoker or if you're over the age of thirty. Check with your doctor to find out whether you are a good candidate for an oral contraceptive and if so which kind would be best for you.

When fitted properly and used correctly, the diaphragm can be up to 95 percent effective. Its effectiveness is increased when it's used in conjunction with a spermicidal jelly or foam. It must be fitted by a health-care professional, who will also instruct you on how to use it properly. Although it has no side effects, it does require advance planning and proper insertion before intercourse.

The condom is up to 85 percent effective, particularly when combined with spermicidal jelly or foam. It is also a good barrier to the spread of sexually transmitted disease. Naturally, it requires the cooperation of your male partner.

The IUD (interuterine device) years ago was found to be highly effective, but it carried some health risks, the most notable of which was pelvic inflammatory disease (PID). Because it was suspected of causing pelvic infection, many manufacturers ceased production. Check with your doctor if you're interested in using this method.

Rhythm and withdrawal methods are the least effective techniques and are not recommended for Type I diabetics because of their unreliability. If you're not prepared for pregnancy, don't trust either rhythm or withdrawal.

JUNE AND BARBARA: Maybe it's time to turn to what population experts call the "missing 50 percent of family planning": the men. It would seem that the very best contraceptive for a diabetic woman would be an effective male contraceptive (injection, pill, or implant) for her partner. That way he could contend with the side effects which might be detrimental to her diabetes. What are the developments on that scene? We rather suspect that male doctors and research scientists don't have their hearts in the project.

DR. LOIS: A male contraceptive has not yet been perfected. Perhaps you are right. "It is the woman's responsibility"—so saith the men.

JUNE AND BARBARA: We read recently about a clinical study of a new male contraceptive. Once a week the men have to inject 200 milligrams of testosterone into a thigh muscle with a two-inch needle. It was reported that the injection "kicked like a cranky mule" and that some of the men in the study put on several pounds and/or developed acne. Do you think this contraceptive is likely to catch on?

DR. LOIS: Why not? We women have put up with more!

JUNE AND BARBARA: What if a diabetic woman does not want to *ever* have children? Would a tubal ligation be hazardous?

DR. LOIS: A tubal ligation is not a hazardous procedure and would not be hazardous in the case of a diabetic woman, but I would only recommend it when a woman is absolutely, *positively* certain that she does not want to have children.

JUNE AND BARBARA: Do you ever recommend a vasectomy for the husband?

DR. LOIS: Only when the husband requests it. I would not recommend it to a man on my own. I must admit that I feel confident to counsel a woman, but to extend that kind of advice to a husband—who is not my patient—is overstepping my bounds.

JUNE AND BARBARA: Is there ever a time when you advise a woman not to have children?

DR. LOIS: I do when a woman has diabetic kidney disease. Unfortunately, the statistics today say that after the onset of protein leakage into the urine from a damaged kidney, the patient is destined to be on dialysis within five years. Persons with diabetes do not usually do well on dialysis, and thus at least half of these persons are dead in another five years. With this stark information at hand, when a woman with diabetic kidney disease contemplates pregnancy I reassure her that her chances of having a healthy child are excellent with a program of blood-glucose normalization. However, I let her know that she may not live to see the child start kindergarten.

How does she feel about leaving her husband alone with a small child? Perhaps it is her way of making sure that her husband will not be alone, but will the burden be too great for him to bear? Only the woman can make this decision, not the physician. I can only state the facts in order to help her come to an educated decision.

JUNE AND BARBARA: In answering the questions about sex, you mentioned vaginitis. We hear a lot about that from diabetic women. Are they more susceptible to it than nondiabetic women?

DR. LOIS: Vaginitis is a normal female problem potentiated by diabetes. It's important to remember that with

vaginitis a specific bacteriological *and* microscopic examination must be made. Vaginal discharges may look, feel,
and smell the same, but the culprit bug could be any one
or many from a large list. The only way to treat vaginitis, therefore, is to send some of the secretion to the
laboratory for culture and to examine it under a microscope. There are four classifications of vaginal discharges:

1.  *Normal.* No infection, just a large amount of se-
    cretions.
2.  *Bacterial.* Example: hemophilus, gonorrhea, chla-
    mydia.
3.  *Parasites.* Example: *Trichomonas.*
4.  *Yeast.* Example: *Candida.*

Each of the above organisms requires a different local
care, and some necessitate that oral medication be taken.
Some can actually be the cause of sterility. High blood-
sugar levels can make these infections worse. Without
the appropriate therapy, the infection will never be
cured. Therefore, unless the gynecologist takes a specimen for the laboratory and looks at it personally under
the microscope, the cream prescribed may not be treating the infection at all.

JUNE AND BARBARA: Since some vaginal discharges are
normal and some are not, could you help us distinguish
between the two?

DR. LOIS: Normal vaginal discharge has different characteristics at different times. Early in the menstrual cycle
it is mixed with the menstrual blood. From day five until
day twelve, it is thick and very light yellow. It has a
subtle, musky odor. On the day of ovulation, it becomes

thin and watery, and then by day sixteen or so it is back to thick. It does not itch or stain.

A discharge usually associated with an infection is one that smells foul, has a brown or deep yellow color, may be as thick as cottage cheese, or itches and burns.

**JUNE AND BARBARA:** One woman who has frequent vaginal infections wrote to ask if there is an approved way to collect the discharge and just bring it to the doctor to be cultured; this would save the time of having to go to the doctor with the complaint and then receive instructions on how to collect the sample. She also wondered if there are any home tests for vaginal discharges, just as there are now tests for blood sugar and for blood in the stool.

**DR. LOIS:** There is no quick self-test. The discharge needs to be cultured for at least five kinds of bacteria, one kind of yeast, and one kind of parasite *(Trichomonas)*. And these cultures need to be handled in a special way *immediately* after the specimen is taken, so this answers the first part of your question. The gynecologist can decide which culture to take after looking at the discharge under a microscope. Bacteria are small round circles, yeast looks like budding beads, and a trichomonad is a moving circle with a tail. Expertise takes awhile to acquire, and a home test would therefore be impossible.

**JUNE AND BARBARA:** One woman asked us if there is any douche that is particularly recommended, or *not* recommended, for diabetic women.

**DR. LOIS:** No, one douche over another is not necessarily better for women with diabetes. But the message is that if a woman has a vaginal infection manifested by discharge, odor, staining, or itching, she should seek medical advice. Vaginitis may adversely affect blood-sugar control, and poor blood-sugar control in turn adversely affects vaginitis. Specific medication for the problem is necessary. Over-the-counter douches will *not* cure the infection.

JUNE AND BARBARA: Now let's explore some of the general problems and possibilities of Type I diabetes, those that pertain to Type I women of all ages.

The ideal way of achieving good control would seem to be to test your own blood sugar and adjust your own insulin dose accordingly, but that can be risky if you don't know what you're doing. How can you tell—and how can your *doctor* tell—if you're intelligent and sufficiently educated in diabetes to handle it?

DR. LOIS: Your level of intelligence or formal education, the number of hours you've sat in diabetes classes, or even the number of books you've read on the subject are not the key issues in whether you're able to take on the responsibility of adjusting your own insulin. What is needed is a trial period. During this time, you don't actually change the doses of insulin you take but instead you record a minimum of a week's worth of blood-sugar tests, performed at least four times a day. In going over these records with your health-care professional, you say which blood sugars you felt needed touching up and which insulin adjustments you would have made at the time.

In this way your health-care professional can learn if you're making knowledgeable decisions that indicate a true understanding of how the kinds of insulin you're taking work in your body under different life circumstances. If you make a wrong suggestion, you can be corrected and instructed in the insulin-dosage concept in which you've shown some confusion. All this learning takes place without the chance of your getting into trouble. It's rather like taking a course in investing in which you pretend to buy certain stocks and then see if they go up or down without actually risking real money.

You should not, of course, take over full command of your insulin therapy until you've shown proper judgment in all situations.

**JUNE AND BARBARA:** June's been adjusting her own insulin for the last sixteen years, since she got a meter and was able to see accurately what her blood sugars were. She just kind of eased into a trial-and-error insulin-adjustment program. She did it without formal instruction, which wasn't available then, but it would have been a lot easier—and she probably would have made fewer mistakes—if she'd had a trial period such as the one you suggest. For the woman who's going to follow this trial-period plan, how long would you estimate it would take before she could confidently take over her insulin adjustment?

**DR. LOIS:** Most surveys estimate that it takes about twenty hours of input from a health-care professional before you can expect to master all the skills necessary to take full command of the insulin-adjustment regime. Whether you're a high-school graduate or a Ph.D., it seems to take about the same amount of time.

If, after those twenty hours of intensive input, you still show errors of judgment in insulin dosage, then you shouldn't try to adjust your own insulin. To pick up the investment-class analogy again, if on paper you kept losing thousands and thousands of dollars, then you'd be more than foolish to start investing your hard-earned real money using the same bad judgment.

JUNE AND BARBARA: We all prefer tight blood-sugar control, but aren't there some conditions, such as heart problems, when it's a good idea to have blood sugars a little on the high side? And if so, how high?

DR. LOIS: I can think of two situations in which control needs to be a little looser: a child under the age of seven, or a person with heart disease.

Children under seven do not have the muscle coordination necessary to take full charge of their own diabetes. If a low blood sugar were coming on, they could not take responsibility to check and fix it. Recent psychological studies have shown a connection between severe childhood hypoglycemic episodes and decreased intelligence. This is the danger with tight control.

As I said before, the number of years a child has diabetes before puberty does not play a role in the subsequent development of complications. Therefore, to help the parents and child get a good night's sleep, a rule of thumb would be to give the child a large bedtime snack, even if this caused the blood sugar to be a bit high all night (180–240 mg/dl). As the child reaches puberty (at approximately eight years and up), every attempt should be made to tighten control, because at that point the clock starts ticking toward complications unless blood sugars are normalized.

Now, about those with heart disease: Hypoglycemia is associated with an outpouring of adrenaline. This hormone produces the energy of "fight or flight," which means that the pulse races and the blood pressure and blood sugar go up. If a person has a limited cardiac reserve because of poor blood flow from atherosclerotic coronary-artery disease, the hypoglycemia could lead to a heart attack. Although this event is unlikely, persons with diabetes and atherosclerotic heart disease should maintain blood-glucose levels of above 100 mg/dl.

JUNE AND BARBARA: One of our major missions has always been to spread the word about the dangers of hyperglycemia and to teach diabetic women that high blood sugars can be avoided with the self-knowledge gained through blood-sugar self-testing. We were appalled by people who were willing to run around with blood sugars over 200 and even 300, risking frightening long-range complications.

Now, after years of preaching control of hyperglycemia, we've become aware that hypoglycemia has its own set of dangers.

The following anonymous letter from a young woman is just one of several we've received about the perils of insulin shock:

Have I got a low-blood-sugar story for you! After years (eleven, to be exact) of walking around (or rather dragging around) with extremely high blood sugars, I saw the light and began an intensive management routine of four injections and five to seven blood tests per day. (I was inspired to do this after reading the Peterson/Jovanovic book.) I had always been afraid of hypoglycemia, and I now realize it was because my former therapy involved taking only one whopping shot of long-range insulin (sixty units of NPH) every day. I had never had any dietary counseling and didn't practice any real consistency in meal and snack times. Consequently, the afternoon hypoglycemic "punch" packed by that large dose of NPH was disturbing and extremely un-comfortable. I had assumed that if I went on a multiple-injection program, my blood sugar would be even more precarious, and I'd have that horrible afternoon confusion all of the time.

Imagine my delight when, once I got real control, I discovered that I could function quite well with no symptoms at all, even when my glucose was in the 40–50 range. Cool! Neat!! Free sailing from now on. I then adopted the "lower-the-better" routine. I even tempted fate when exercising. Even though I had precalibrated my favorite remedy (five jelly beans = 30 mg rise in blood sugar), I hesitated to take it, for when I got home from exercising, wouldn't it be better to record a 60 in my diary rather than a 90?

One evening in early December, I got home from work feeling tense and knew I wanted to take a walk around one of Minneapolis's beautiful inner-city lakes (about three miles). The temperature was five degrees above zero, but being a native Minnesotan, I was prepared with adequate clothing. I took two fewer units than usual of regular insu-lin, ate my usual supper featuring 50 grams of carbohy-drate, packed my jelly beans, and set out.

The jogging path where I usually walk is consistently heavily populated, so I had no qualms about going out by myself, even though it was dark. When I reached the lake, however, the path was slick with ice, and I decided to walk the perimeter on a sidewalk a few hundred feet away, on the edge of a residential section (dark and *un*populated).

I also realized it was a lot colder than I'd anticipated (with the wind chill, which I hadn't bothered to check, it was actually –45°). Probably due to the fact that I was using a lot of calories to keep warm, I began to feel light-headed after about twenty minutes of walking, yet I stubbornly re-fused to eat the sugar. After about twenty more minutes, I was barely able to think clearly, so I reached for the beans, only to find them frozen solid.

By that time, it was too late anyway, and I fell headfirst into a snowbank. It was simply luck that a passing pedestrian saw me tumble. If I had fallen when no one was around, I probably wouldn't have been discovered until the next morning, either dead as a doornail or severely frostbitten.

I am tempted to chuckle about this incident, for I feel humor is a very useful tool, but it's not all that funny. In fact, it is so embarrassing that I am declining to sign my name to this.

What would I suggest after this happened to me? To never exercise alone? Of course not. But be prepared, don't take chances, and keep in mind that one's life is more important than "perfect" numbers in one's blood-sugar diary.

Even if it had been light out and had not been during winter, I probably would not have carried my meter or strips with me. I justify this because it is difficult enough for me to interrupt my normal daily routine to make the tests, and I don't want to drag all that stuff around during my leisure time. But I was reasonably sure that hypoglycemia was setting in, and like a fool I persisted anyway.

Has this incident changed my way of thinking? Not really. I need to remind myself of this near miss often and to also keep in mind that if I do overshoot with the sugar, I now have the tools to bring my blood glucose down to normal range with an extra squirt of Regular.

Some things will no doubt take me a lifetime to figure out, but I would still advise anyone taking a single injection per day to give multiples a try. This system has afforded me more flexibility and dietary freedom than I ever thought possible, not to mention "euglycemia." (I love that term.)

P.S. I now carry the jelly beans in a pocket next to my body, where they stay close to body temperature.

This story—and others like it—put us in mind of one of James Thurber's *Fables for Our Time*, "The Bear Who Let It Alone."

Thurber described a hard-drinking bear who would reel home at night, knock down the lamps, ram his elbows through windows, and then collapse on the floor and fall asleep. His wife was distressed, and his children were very frightened.

Then, suddenly, the bear reformed and became a famous teetotaler. He told everybody who came to the house how strong and well he had become since he stopped drinking. To prove it, he would stand on his head and on his hands and turn cartwheels, knocking down the lamps and ramming his elbows through windows. Then, tired by his healthy exercise, he would lie down on the floor and go to sleep. His wife was distressed, and his children were very frightened.

Moral: YOU MIGHT AS WELL FALL FLAT ON YOUR FACE AS LEAN OVER TOO FAR BACKWARD.

It is admittedly difficult to walk the euglycemic tightrope of perfect control without toppling off from time to time. Is there *any* way you can be sure of never having a hypoglycemic reaction? June still has them on occasion. Are you, yourself, able to avoid them entirely?

DR. LOIS: When a person has a blood-glucose level of 200–300 mg/dl all the time, she has plenty of room to fall—even as much as 100 points at a time. But when you keep your blood sugar in the recommended range of around 100 and if each unit of insulin can bring the blood glucose down 25 points, then an overcalculation of two units of insulin, or a matching undercalculation of twenty grams of carbohydrate, can result in bad hypoglycemia if the blood-glucose level falls much below 100 mg/dl. Sometimes a bit more exercise than usual can precipitate a hypoglycemic reaction.

Sure, I could prevent hypoglycemic reactions by *never* having a blood sugar below 200 mg/dl, but then I am at greater risk for complications of diabetes. The solution is to be prepared. Pocket food and desk-drawer juices are ever present.

Even with all that, yes, I have been caught unaware when I was terribly distracted by a busy work schedule and have drifted into never-never land. Yes, it *is* embarrassing, but every time I make a blooper it makes me more determined to try harder to prevent these occurrences. In one case I passed out at a dinner party because the service was poor. (Ironically, this was a party at the National Diabetes Association Meeting, and fifty of the most prominent diabetologists in America seemed more prone to panic than to coming to my rescue!) Another time I was in an airplane so small that the hand luggage was put into the nose of the plane and I couldn't get to my food supply. I became so low I had a convulsion and ended up in the emergency room of a Detroit hospital.

I certainly don't like to admit my bloopers, but if I can learn from my mistakes to prevent another such episode in myself as well as in my patients, then it's worth retelling the experiences.

JUNE AND BARBARA: A serious problem that has developed with the onset of tight control is what's called "hypoglycemic unawareness." It seems to trouble almost half the people with long-standing diabetes; at least that's what happened in the DCCT study. These people had lost their natural protections that keep blood sugar normal. These are the release of glucagon, a pancreatic hormone that raises blood sugar, and epinephrine (adrenaline), which tells you you're low with symptoms such as shaking and perspiring.

John Walsh, author of *The Pocket Pancreas*, points out another important piece of information. "Having one insulin reaction increases the risk for another: In one study, 46 percent of people who had a reaction had another reaction the same day, 24 percent on the second day, and 12 percent on the third day. Unfortunately, the second reaction is harder to recognize because stress hormones, which create symptoms like sweating and shaking, are largely depleted by the first reaction for the next two or three days."

We deduce from all this that it's a good idea to try very hard to keep your insulin reactions to a minimum by checking your blood sugar more frequently or even in some cases by allowing your average blood sugar to be somewhat higher. In fact, studies suggest that hypoglycemic unawareness may be reversible and the release of glucagon and epinephrine normalized after three months of meticulous prevention of all hypoglycemia.

We shouldn't leave this subject without telling you that it's vital for every insulin-taking diabetic to keep glucagon on hand. This hormone raises blood sugar rapidly by causing glucose stored in the liver to be released. Glucagon can be injected just like insulin in cases of severe hypoglycemia. It is available in pharmacies by prescription in a convenient Glucagon Emergency Kit made by Eli Lilly. Make sure a family member or friend is instructed in exactly how to inject it and, equally important, where to find it!

To turn to the other end of the blood-sugar scale, many women complain of frequently waking up with high blood sugars when they had been normal the night before. Some of them have been told that they have "Somogiied" in the night or that they've experienced the "dawn phenomenon." Could you explain what these two are?

DR. LOIS: Somogii is a hypoglycemic episode that takes place around three in the morning. You sleep through it, and it is associated with the following:

1. Having a bad dream
2. Waking up with a low temperature
3. Waking up with high blood sugar as a compensatory response to the low blood sugar
4. Waking up with ketones in the urine from using fat breakdown to bring up the low blood sugar

Dr. Somogii was a Hungarian who described this phenomenon in 1956 and claimed it was due to an overdose of the morning NPH; his name was given to this syndrome. Technically, a low at 3 A.M. from bedtime NPH or regular cannot be called Somogii, although the wake-up high blood sugar is caused by the same compensatory mechanisms.

Since I try to be a purist, I use the word *bounce* to describe the phenomenon of a low followed three hours later by a high. When blood sugar is low, it signals adrenaline (epinephrine and norepinephrine), glucagon, growth hormone, and cortisol (in that order) to pour out and go to the liver and break down glycogen to produce sugar. The liver pours out sugar over the next three hours, and the result is usually a very high blood sugar.

Then there's what's known as the dawn phenomenon. The wake-up hormones, cortisol and growth hormone, rise with the sun. These hormones provide the trigger that gets us up to go in the morning. They are also anti-insulin in nature in that they make the action of insulin weaker. The blood sugar will rise if more insulin is not taken. This rise of the morning blood sugar between 3 and 9 A.M. is called the dawn phenomenon.

If a 3 A.M. low happens, the four stress hormones mentioned above will add to the two wake-up hormones to cause the blood sugar to bounce even higher.

Whether you feel your problem is Somogii or the dawn phenomenon, the strategy for avoiding high wake-up blood sugar is the same. You must prevent the 3 A.M. blood sugar from dropping below 70 mg/dl and you must have extra insulin available from 4 A.M. onward.

The ways to avoid dropping below 70 around 3 A.M. are to increase your bedtime snack or to decrease your evening long-acting insulin (NPH, lente or ultralente). For those on a pump, decrease your bedtime basal. To control the 4 A.M. rise, switch your before-dinner injection of long-acting insulin to a before-bedtime injection (this delays the peaking and may coincide better with your wake-up hormones). If on a pump, add more insulin to the basal rate after 4 A.M.

JUNE AND BARBARA: Since it's often a battle to keep blood sugars normal, we get many questions asking what new therapies are available to help win that battle. Fortunately, there are more new treatments every day, including jet-injection therapy and the pump. We'll describe jets, because June has three different generations of them, dating from 1985 and let you do pumps, since your experience with them goes back to 1981.

Using a jet injector is about the only way to take insulin without using a needle. With a jet, the insulin itself becomes a needle because it is shot with jetlike speed. All you feel is nothing or something like snapping your finger against your skin. If you suffer from needle phobia, these needleless injectors are about the only answer for you. But we think their advantages go way beyond that. Most important, they disperse the insulin under your skin in a spray and therefore you get more uniform absorption and more predictable and consistent control of your blood sugar.

This is not to say that jet injectors are any kind of panacea. Some who use them get pain-free, bruise-free injections while others have problems. They are also fairly expensive—between $600 and $700 at present—and require a doctor's prescription. Most of the manufacturers have a thirty-day trial period, and a video is supplied for instruction. The two most experienced manufacturers are Medi-Ject Corporation, 1840 Berkshire Lane, Minneapolis, MN 55441 (1-800-328-3074) and Vitajet Corporation, 27075 Cabot Rd., #102, Laguna Hills, CA 92653 (1-800-848-2538). Here are illustrations of two of the current models:

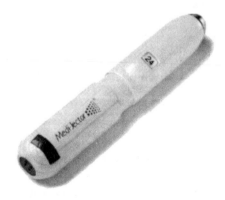

*Figure 1a*    Medi-jector

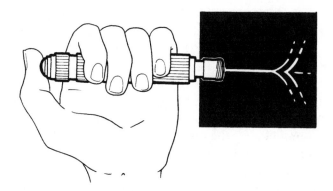

*Figure 1b* VitaPen

Now, Dr. Lois, why don't you tell us about pumps including your own personal experiences with one.

**DR. LOIS:** Perhaps I should first describe a pump so that everyone will know exactly what we're talking about. An insulin-infusion pump is a battery-operated portable box that houses a syringe with at least a day's supply of insulin. The pump slowly pushes the plunger of the syringe so that insulin flows through a long tube that has a needle attached to the end. The needle is placed under the skin, usually in the abdomen, and is taped in place. The needle stays in place for one to three days and is then replaced by a new one. There is also a way to take out the needle and leave behind a small plastic tube, and this is more comfortable.

The amount of insulin infused over the whole day (twenty-four hours) is called the basal rate. The basal rate is defined as that amount of insulin that keeps a Type I diabetic person normoglycemic (that is, with blood sugar always in the normal range) when she is not eating. When she wishes to eat, she simply pushes a button on the box to increase the dose of insulin to cover the meal. Only regular insulin is put into the syringe.

Usually the basal rate is calculated to be 0.3 times the weight of the person in kilograms. The overnight basal tends to be different from the daytime basal. From midnight until 4 A.M., the rate is usually 0.2 times the weight in kilograms, and from 4 A.M. to 10 A.M. it is usually 0.4 times the weight in kilograms. Once again, each person is different, so blood-glucose self-monitoring must be performed and the rate changed accordingly in order to derive the right basal rates.

The mealtime increased insulin need is about one unit of regular for every 10 grams of carbohydrate in the meal to be eaten at lunch and dinner. Breakfast tends to need more insulin due to the dawn phenomenon. The ratio at breakfast is 1.5 units for each ten grams of carbohydrate. This extra injection of Regular (called the bolus) needs to be given far enough ahead of the meal so that the insulin and the food meet the bloodstream at the same moment.

Each person must derive her own lag time by starting a meal with a blood sugar of between 70 and 100 mg/dl, taking one unit of Regular for every 10 grams of carbohydrate in the meal to be eaten, and then checking blood sugar every fifteen minutes. When the blood sugar has dropped by 15 mg/dl, the meal can be eaten. The amount of time between the injection of the extra Regular and the blood sugar's fall to 15 mg/dl is the lag time. This is the amount of time that must always elapse before you eat a meal.

JUNE AND BARBARA: For which types of diabetics do you recommend the pump?

DR. LOIS: Pumps are not for everyone. Many patients have stable blood-glucose levels on only one or two injections a day. A pump would not improve control. It would only make diabetes care more complicated.

In cases in which good glucose control can only be achieved with three or more injections a day, the pump can make the process of self-care a bit more convenient. A woman must earn her pump, however. If she is not willing to perform blood-glucose self-monitoring at least four times a day, she is not responsible enough to have an insulin pump. To keep the pump safe, at least four blood-sugar tests a day are necessary.

JUNE AND BARBARA: Now that we know what a pump is and how it works, tell us about your own experience with it.

DR. LOIS: Fifteen years ago I was very much antipump. I was bigoted enough to believe that control equal to that on an insulin pump could be achieved with numerous injections. Personally, however, I was having a terrible time on three injections a day of NPH and Regular. Some days I would be high in the afternoon, and some days I would have a bad insulin reaction in the afternoon. Begrudgingly, I tried a pump.

Now, this was in the old days, when the pump was HUGE! The pump certainly smoothed out my afternoon dilemma, but I paid a dear price. I had to wear the "badge of courage." None of my clothes worked with a pump—certainly, none of my pretty clothes did. In addition, people thought of me as sick. "What is *that?*" they would ask. "Is it a life-support machine?"

And never mind the airport-security guards who ripped the pump off my belt to examine it better, pulling my needle out in the process!

Then there was the fear of sleeping alone. Of course all Type I diabetics have that fear to a certain extent, but wearing the pump exacerbated these fears. The reports of overnight hypoglycemia attacks had even *me* scared. Since I travel frequently, I am often alone in a hotel room, so I soon learned to pack provisions along with all my pump gear. Having to be dependent on an electrical outlet to keep my batteries charged also decreased my flexibility in traveling abroad.

In the total picture, I am not sure that the problems of wearing a huge pump didn't outweigh any advantages.

But then along came the "baby" pumps. These pumps could be easily hidden in even my prettiest clothes. The batteries now lasted two to three months, and I could get more flexibility in programming various basal rates. What a delight! My pump blues are gone—well, *almost* gone—now that I wear a small pump. I still have skin problems if I keep a needle in place even a teeny bit too long, and the tubing is still expensive. But I no longer feel like a freakish person in a crowd, carrying around my big black box.

JUNE AND BARBARA: It's very encouraging how pumps are constantly being improved to make them easier to use. The two manufacturers are MiniMed (1-800-933-3322, extension 3463) and Disetronic (1-800-280-7801). Both companies are constantly making changes for the better in their pumps. Check with them for the latest developments. For in-depth information on pumps, there are now two basic books: *Pumping Insulin*, by John Walsh and Ruth Roberts, and *The Insulin Pump Therapy Book*, edited by Linda Fredrickson. (See Basic Books on Diabetes in Appendix A: Recommended Reading.)

In the last nine years, there have been many other

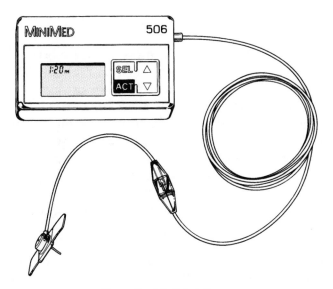

*Figure 2*   MiniMed Pump

technological advances on all fronts. We've heard that approximately forty-four different companies are working on a "noninvasive" blood-sugar test that can be done without puncturing your finger to get a drop of blood (using infrared beams, skin patches, etc.). Additionally, there's talk of a GlucoWatch with a pad adhering to the skin, which measures blood sugar transdermally (through the skin) that is supposed to provide a continuous readout. Could you give us some hints and hopes about such advances and especially some late information about the possibilities of a cure?

DR. LOIS: Although the "sugar watch" is not ready for the marketplace, the keen competition and the financial rewards of such may mean that by the year 2000 we shall have one. If I had to guess, I think the Japanese will win this race.

Although oral insulin will probably never become a treatment, it is becoming a prevention. Research has suggested that if a person is found to be predisposed to developing diabetes by a test called "anti-islet cell antibodies," then drinking insulin may trick the immune system into not destroying the person's pancreas. When insulin is drunk, it is denatured by gastric juices, and the small pieces that absorb do not affect the blood sugar but they do fool the immune system.

As for a cure, instead of pancreas transplants, encapsulating the pancreatic insulin-producing islet cells has taken the lead. Here the research has exploded, thank goodness. There are three types of capsules to protect the insulin-secreting cells, so that when they are implanted in your body they can be protected against rejection. There are 1) spheres put into the blood stream; 2) polymers surrounding the cells and then the cells injected into the abdominal space; and 3) tubes with cells implanted under the skin, much like the birth-control devices now available.

JUNE AND BARBARA: We need to ask about a special insulin problem that's very close to home (June has it) and that seems to affect more people than was originally thought. While it's true that doctors—we assume—now routinely put all their patients on the synthetic human insulins made since 1982 by the two major insulin companies in the U.S., Lilly and Novo Nordisk, many long-term diabetics have continued to use animal insulins from pig and cow pancreases and have been well controlled with them. These animal insulins also used to be less expensive.

Then, wham-o, the two drug companies started pulling animal insulin off the market and a certain percentage of people, forced to switch, found they couldn't retain good control on human insulins. Some suffered unrecognizable insulin reactions and others uncustomary high blood sugars. Dangerous and frustrating. Over the last decade, in spite of some studies claiming no culpability for the synthetics, the debate has continued, especially in Britain, where in 1995 the British Diabetic Association collected 140,000 signatures on a petition urging drug companies to provide animal insulins indefinitely.

We understand the British plea perfectly. June had been on Novo Nordisk beef ultralente for over fifteen years, and she got big swings in her blood sugar in 1994 after the company took it off the market and she tried Lilly human ultralente (for the second time, as she had experimented with it when it first arrived on the scene). In desperation she then switched to Novo's human Lente, next to their human NPH, and finally to their purified pork NPH and that did it, but the pork insulin has become hard to find and much more expensive. What to do? Are June and her sister-travelers simply more animal than human and condemned to an experimental existence?

DR. LOIS: Animal insulins may be available someday for "compassionate" use. Drug companies many times place money into drugs that are only used in a small population. These drugs are nicknamed "orphan drugs," because they usually do not have a parent company to market them. Producing an "orphan drug" is excellent public relations for a company and can be effectively used to promote public satisfaction with them for their humanitarianism. Perhaps animal insulin will be Lilly's or Novo Nordisk's orphan drug.

JUNE AND BARBARA: Another problem with insulin is with its absorption. We know that jets improve absorption and we've also read that pumps provide more predictability, while needles can alter absorption by as much as 10 to 50 percent of the daily injected dose. Dr. Philip Raskin in *The Insulin Pump Therapy Book* reports that "variable insulin absorption is responsible for up to 80 percent of the day-to-day flluctuations in blood-glucose concentrations in persons using injection-based therapy." How do you know whether you have this problem and what can you do about it?

DR. LOIS: If you inject the right amount of insulin to cover the meal you're going to eat and afterward your blood sugar rises for no apparent reason, then it's likely that the insulin did not absorb on schedule. My rule of thumb in that case is never to inject in that spot again. Absorption is slowed when the injection is made in a place where marks have been made by numerous insulin injections.

Absorption is *always* affected by the site of injection. Different areas on the body absorb insulin at different rates. Usually, the skin on the lower abdomen absorbs the fastest. There are several tricks you can perform to increase the absorption rate of insulin. After injecting the insulin, exercise the muscles where the injection was made. If you inject into the arm, do push-ups; if you inject in the leg, do knee-bends or jumping jacks. In addition, applying heat with a warm washcloth and/or vigorously rubbing the area of injection can increase absorption rates. Injection of insulin directly into muscle speeds up absorption by twenty minutes. I suggest using the calf muscle and then doing jumping jacks.

JUNE AND BARBARA: The older unpurified insulins caused fat atrophy (lipoatrophy) for many women. The signs of such atrophy are the canyons and caverns that appear where insulin is repeatedly injected. Antibodies that your body produces in response to the beef/pork and beef insulins can gobble up fat cells at the injection site. This is not a pleasant state of affairs for anyone, but for young women who want to appear in shorts and bathing suits, it's particularly distressing.

We also heard from a young woman lawyer who's now happily back in bathing suits that if you shoot human insulin into the canyons and caverns, they may well fill in so you'll look as smooth as before. Have you found this to be the case, or do you think this woman's fat atrophy filled in for a different reason?

DR. LOIS: Yes, the depressions caused by years of insulin injections with beef/pork insulin will eventually fill in if the highly purified insulins are injected first at the edges of the depressions. Then, as they fill in, the injections can be given closer and closer to the center of the depression.

JUNE AND BARBARA: Another woman had the opposite problem. She was worried because she had always injected into her thighs and had developed such large bumps at the injection sites that she could no longer wear shorts or pants that fit snugly. What should she do?

DR. LOIS: To minimize "bumps" at injections sites, smaller doses of insulin should be injected. Her diabetes team can help her plan three to four injections a day. In addition, she should switch to buffered Regular insulin (the bottle says BR). I would also recommend that she inject in her abdomen. She should ask her diabetes nurse specialist to double-check her technique. After all, if she learned to inject insulin when she was a little girl, it may be that she made bumps because of the way she was injecting.

JUNE AND BARBARA: Another insulin prejudice we have is that we don't think anybody can have good therapy on only one shot of NPH a day. Is this true?

DR. LOIS: Almost, but not quite. Diabetic women who still have some pancreatic function can get along on only one shot of NPH. The way they can check themselves for this is to see whether they always have normal fasting blood sugars. If they do, then this one-shot insulin therapy is all right for them. But no Type I diabetic without pancreatic function—and this is the vast majority—can possibly achieve optimum control with one shot of NPH a day.

JUNE AND BARBARA: Mercifully, it's a lot more convenient now to take multiple shots than it used to be. June is on what is sometimes called "the poor man's pump," but here we'll make that the poor woman's pump. She takes multiple injections: NPH morning and evening, Regular before each meal and whenever her blood sugar needs a little downward fine-tuning. All these injections used to be a drag before the convenience of penlike injection devices. These are used with prefilled insulin cartridges (available in Regular, NPH, and 70/30 premixed insulin). This makes measuring and injecting a quick-

and-easy and unobtrusive matter. With an insulin pen, you always have your insulin with you and ready to go. There are currently two insulin pens available.

The Autopen is made by Owen Mumford, Inc., 849 Pickens Industrial Drive, Suite 14, Marietta, GA 30062-3165, phone: (800) 421-6936. This has a dial-a-dose selector and you see on the dial what dose you're getting or, for those with visual problems or if you're injecting in a poorly illuminated area, you can count the number of clicks. There are two models: one that gives two to thirty-two units in two-unit increments and, for those on a lower dose, one that gives 1 to 16 units in one-unit increments. The Autopen uses Novolin insulin cartridges and needles. Cartridges are available in three formulations of human insulin: Regular, NPH, and 70/30 (70 percent NPH/30 percent Regular).

The Novolin Pen is sold by Novo Nordisk Pharmaceuticals, Inc., 100 Overlook Center, Suite 200, Princeton, NJ 08540, phone: (800) 727-6500. It delivers insulin in two-unit increments and uses Novolin insulin cartridges (see above) and needles.

Novo Nordisk Pharmaceuticals also has developed a prefilled disposable syringe which comes in the same three formulations as the cartridges: Regular, NPH, and 70/30. Each syringe contains 150 units of insulin and delivers up to 58 units per injection in two-unit increments.

Here's a puzzling little ketone adventure based on June's personal experience. She was in Hawaii and got what was either food poisoning or the two-day flu. She treated it with Sugarfree 7-Up and chicken-noodle soup. During the sick period her blood sugars were all perfect—around 100—yet she had ketones. Can you explain why?

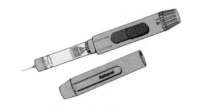

*Figure 3a*    Autopen

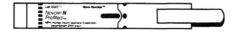

*Figure 3b*    Novolin Prefilled
© 1995 Novo Nordisk Pharmaceuticals Inc.

**DR. LOIS:** Fat cells break down as a normal compensatory mechanism after all the sugar stores have been used up during fasting states. It takes about eighteen hours of fasting to use up the normal fuel stores of sugar, or glycogen, in the liver before fat begins to break down. Fat breakdown results in release of free fatty acids, which go to the liver and are metabolized there to ketone bodies. These ketones can be used by the brain as an alternative fuel source when sugar is used up.

June's illness, which resulted in almost no food intake but an increase in caloric expenditure due to the extra energy used when one has a fever, resulted in fat breakdown to provide her brain with necessary energy.

Fat will also break down spontaneously when the blood levels of insulin are absent or are very low. This is not a case of starvation ketosis, which happens to everyone, but rather of a person with Type I diabetes who has not taken sufficient insulin. Then there is a massive fat breakdown and a massive buildup of free fatty acids, which leads to ketoacidosis.

By the way, children and pregnant women need to fast for only six hours before they use up their liver glycogen and start to break down their fat stores. This is called accelerated starvation. Thus, in times of famine, saving the food for the pregnant women and the children was a very good idea.

JUNE AND BARBARA: One of the unfortunate side effects of the women's movement is that women, especially young women, are drinking and smoking more. Let's take drinking first. Naturally, we know that drinking to excess is not even under consideration, but how about an occasional cocktail or glass of wine? What's the harm in that if there are no other contraindications?

DR. LOIS: Alcohol seems to make insulin stronger, and it usually has its strongest potentiating effect four to six hours after drinking. If alcohol is consumed before bed, the potentiation may occur from 3 to 4 A.M., the very time when the overnight NPH or ultralente tends to lower the blood-sugar level. So I usually ask my diabetic women patients to restrict their evening drinking to one glass of wine and to make sure that their bedtime snack is large enough to prevent a 3 A.M. low.

If more than one glass of wine is drunk, then I ask the woman to take only one-half of her usual dose of NPH and still eat a large bedtime snack.

As you can see, it's easier not to drink at all rather than to second-guess the body's ability to handle the alcohol. Drinking is especially problematic when the drink also has a high sugar content. I usually dip a chem-strip into wine before drinking it to ensure that the wine is not overly sweet. By the way, I test diet sodas with a chemstrip if I think I may have been served the wrong drink. Regular Coca-Cola and 7-UP turn the stick to 800 mg/dl; diet drinks stay at 0.

JUNE AND BARBARA: In every book we've written, we've unleashed a tirade on the evils of smoking. We feel that no woman—in fact no animal, vegetable, or mineral—should ever smoke, under any circumstance. Do you agree?

DR. LOIS: Definitely. Smoking is strongly linked to vascular problems, heart disease, and cancer, but for a diabetic person it has another terrifying consequence. At least 90 percent—and maybe closer to 99 percent—of diabetic people who need amputations are smokers. The good news is that five years on the wagon can reverse this risk.

JUNE AND BARBARA: We once heard one of your colleagues, Dr. Douglas Muchmore of the Scripps Clinic, say, "I advise all of my patients who smoke to quit. For my diabetic patients, I *insist* on it."

DR. LOIS: I agree.

JUNE AND BARBARA: How about marijuana? We know the basic problems that it causes for everyone, but does it also cause special problems with diabetes control?

DR. LOIS: The studies on what marijuana does to blood sugars are equivocal. Most studies say that if a patient does not eat uncontrollably, as with "the munchies," then marijuana has no effect on the blood sugar.

JUNE AND BARBARA: How about other drugs, such as cocaine and heroin?

DR. LOIS: No systematic studies on other illicit drugs have been performed, but I can't imagine why a diabetic woman would needlessly further complicate an already complicated life with drugs—not even on a one-time experimental basis.

JUNE AND BARBARA: Of course there are other drugs, legal drugs, that are taken for physical conditions. How can these affect blood sugar?

DR. LOIS: The following are drugs that don't mix well with diabetes or that may require readjustment of the insulin dosage:

1. *Hypertension medicines.* Diuretics raise the blood sugars. Beta blockers keep the body from releasing its own sugar in response to hypoglycemia.
2. *Arthritis medications.* Both steroids and nonsteroidal anti-inflammatory drugs raise the blood sugar.
3. *Seizure medications.* Phenhydantoin raises blood sugar.
4. *Cold remedies.* Unless they are sugar free, cough syrups raise blood sugar, as do decongestants containing neosynephrine and aphedrine.

JUNE AND BARBARA: You mentioned steroids. When June was having a foot problem, the podiatrist injected cortisone, saying that it "probably would have no effect on her blood sugar." Wrong! Her blood sugars went so high that she had to increase her insulin by half. A young diabetic woman we know was given cortisone for a knee problem, and she had to more than *double* her insulin.

I don't know if there are many diabetic women athletes out there who might be tempted to take steroids to build muscles the way some male athletes do, but if there are, would that have the same effect on their diabetes? Have you heard of any reports on this?

DR. LOIS: I'm happy to say that I have never heard of a diabetic woman trying to build up muscles with steroids—and I hope I never do! If a woman did such a thing she would have to approximately double her usual dose of insulin to avoid high blood sugars. After two days of twice her normal dosage of insulin, she would find it would take another three days for the dosage to fall back to normal. For medical and ethical reasons, I would never prescribe steroids for any of my patients to use for improving their athletic capability. I would hope that most other physicians agree with me.

JUNE AND BARBARA: Do you have any positive tips for women athletes?

DR. LOIS: I would, of course, suggest that they take frequent blood sugars, since either hyperglycemia or hypoglycemia impairs athletic performance. Just as with Bill Carlson, the diabetic triathlete, the pump works well for some ballerinas—who are, in a very real sense, athletes—because they can disconnect it during practice periods and performances when they're exercising heavily.

JUNE AND BARBARA: Speaking of exercise, since a diabetic shouldn't be sedentary, let's all stand up and stretch, do a little running in place, or even take a walk around the block before we move onward and upward into *le deuxième âge*.

# Le Deuxième Age

Calling this period in a woman's life the second age is particularly appropriate, because during these years a second is about all the time you have for yourself—if that! This period is also sometimes known as the "sandwich years," because you're often sandwiched between the demands and responsibilities of your young children and those of your aging parents, and everyone is trying to take a bite out of your time and energy.

The stresses of handling a career and/or marriage and/or motherhood, plus the built-in stresses of dealing with diabetes every day, can be almost overwhelming. You need to be aware of stress and learn how to handle it. (For books on stress reduction, see Recommended Reading: Emotional Health and Stress.)

And yet, as stress expert Hans Selye says, "Stress is the spice of life." These most stressful times are also very exciting times. If you can bring yourself to think of them as exciting rather than stressful, it will make them easier to accept and to cope with.

Since the excitement of giving birth is for most women a peak experience—and one that, until recent years, has been regarded as, if not impossible, then at least very risky and unadvisable for the woman diabetic—we'll devote the lioness's share of this chapter to pregnancy. Here we will explain the new discoveries and therapies that give a woman diabetic the same highly favorable prognosis as a nondiabetic woman for giving birth to a healthy baby.

JUNE AND BARBARA: In one letter a woman gave voice to a problem that is probably common to all women embarking on a career or applying for a new job: "I still felt awkward about listing diabetes on a job application, especially when there is no particular place to list it. Do you feel it is better to mention it during a job interview, when you will have more time for a full explanation of how you control your diabetes? Sometimes the only question on a preliminary job application is 'Do you have any condition which will interfere with your ability to fulfill this job?' Would you ever mention diabetes in a résumé?"

DR. LOIS: No. If I am qualified for a job, my diabetes should not be a reason to disqualify me. Unfortunately, an element of prejudice may creep into decisions about my qualifications if I mention my diabetes.

My diabetes is as private as my fibrocystic breast disease. Unless I am asked point-blank, I do not offer my health problems. Only such jobs as being a pilot or doing construction work on tall buildings would require that an applicant bring up diabetes.

JUNE AND BARBARA: Here's one of those famous bad news, good news situations. The bad news is that you have diabetes, and the good news is that it may make for marital happiness.

At the Southern Illinois University School of Medicine, researchers were surprised and happy to learn that a disease as serious as diabetes could have a positive side. Despite the potential for conflict in the marriages of diabetics, the divorce and separation rate of a group of diabetic patients was relatively low. Only 21 percent had ended their marriages, compared to 46.6 percent among the general population.

Furthermore, a study reported in the *New York Times* found that "seriously ill women are more often than not blessed with loving husbands . . . marriage to such a woman means providing enormous support, and these marriages either founder or are very stable. . . . Marriages to sick women are different—there's more communication. . . . From poor men without jobs to bank presidents, these husbands have thought through their relationships carefully and are extremely loyal." This puts us in mind of Lee Iacocca, who, despite all the pressures of his high-powered work, was always tremendously caring and supportive of his diabetic wife.

Have you noticed this happy situation in your patients, and do you have any other insights as to why this is so?

**DR. LOIS:** Perhaps the answer is that only special men choose wives with diabetes. It is as though they know we are not perfect but still find joy in the talents we have developed to compensate for our affliction.

**JUNE AND BARBARA:** We all know that diabetes runs in families, so one of the first questions a diabetic woman has when contemplating pregnancy is whether or not she will pass diabetes on to her child.

**DR. LOIS:** Yes, there is a chance that diabetes can be passed on to the child, but the chances are less than 6 percent for someone with Type I diabetes. If you have Type II diabetes, the risk of passing it on to the child may rise to 25 percent. If you have gestational diabetes, it is possible that your daughters will also have gestational diabetes, and you yourself have a 60 percent chance of developing Type II diabetes.

Remember that babies are *not* born with diabetes. It usually occurs at eight to fourteen years of age. A rule of thumb is that if your child has inherited your genetic tendency to have diabetes and comes in contact with the "environmental trigger," then she or he will probably get diabetes at the same age that you did.

JUNE AND BARBARA: On the subject of having children, one of our oldest friends is Sharon, a former diabetes nurse-educator who presented us with an interesting situation. She is a diabetic woman with many complications, including diabetic retinopathy, which requires laser treatments. Sharon and her husband, Glenn, agreed that because of her many health problems it would be better for them not to have any children. Fortunately, this decision has not caused them great personal anguish, since Glenn had never particularly wanted to have children anyway and it was thus not a major issue. However, they do have a problem with other people (as Sartre said, "Hell is other people"). On discovering that Sharon and Glenn have no children, many people seem disturbed. When, after cooing something like, "Well, when are you and your husband going to start your little family?" they learn that the couple has no intention of having children, they are aghast.

Sharon became so tired of this that she started telling people that her doctor had absolutely forbidden her to become pregnant. This seemed to work, but Sharon said that she felt guilty laying the blame on the doctor when actually it was her and Glenn's decision (although the doctor did agree that their decision was a sound one). It was our opinion that Sharon should go ahead with what she was doing. We felt that it was nobody's business but hers and that the doctor probably wouldn't mind being implicated if he ever found out.

DR. LOIS: I agree with your opinion that it's okay to ease the psychological burden of making a hard decision by sharing the decision making, or, in this case, the "blame," with the physician. I particularly remember one case of actual shared decision making that may illustrate this philosophy.

I was asked to advise a woman about whether or not she should have a therapeutic abortion. She had a glycosylated-hemoglobin level of 14 percent (more than twice the normal level), and she had been told that the risk of having a child with a birth defect was 20 to 30 percent. This also meant that she had a 70 to 80 percent chance of having a normal child. She was in terrible conflict and felt terribly guilty about wanting to abort.

I sensed this woman's ambivalence and distress over having to make this choice, yet I also sensed that she did not want to have a defective child if the risk was so high. Taking my cues from her, I took the responsibility and told her that if it were *my* decision I would abort, get myself into super diabetes control, and then start over to have a perfect baby. I therefore recommended that she undergo an abortion. Diabetic women usually have only one or two chances to bear children, and it would be a shame to invest time, energy, and money in a poor start.

This woman's depression lifted immediately. She felt relieved that she did not have to be the one to make such a decision. Her physician had told her what to do.

But, of course, I was listening to her soul when I advised her and recommended to her that she do what she didn't have the courage to do alone. Had her soul told me that she wanted this baby, no matter what, I would have told her to keep the child.

So you see, shared blame is okay.

**JUNE AND BARBARA:** You mentioned earlier that it's not advisable for a woman on dialysis to get pregnant. What if she has a successful kidney transplant? Would that make it all right?

DR. LOIS: Nine years ago when we wrote the first edition of this book, I wasn't able to answer this question because kidney transplantation for people with diabetes had only been available for ten years. During that period only a handful of diabetic women with kidney transplants had had pregnancies. Although these women, their kidneys, and their babies had done well, I felt we needed more experience before I could say that all would be well after a kidney transplant.

Happily, the last nine years have shown that kidney-transplant patients do very well during pregnancy. In fact, most kidney specialists recommend a transplant before a pregnancy in a woman with end-stage kidney disease. The babies do very well if the diabetes and kidney disease are both treated before pregnancy.

JUNE AND BARBARA: In an article in the *New York Times*, "Having Children Despite Illness," the author, Jane Gross, explores the motivation behind the decision of chronically ill women to have children.

Interviews with a half dozen chronically ill women and their doctors indicate that they are largely motivated by a desire to be normal, to test the body that has so often failed them, to be like everyone else.

"When your pancreas doesn't work, there's the feeling that you're defective," said Donna Jornsay, a diabetic mother with a one-year-old daughter. "The desire to prove the rest of you works is absolutely compelling. Also, you're confronted with your own mortality so much sooner than other people, and the desire to see some piece of you live on is very strong."

Do you see these motivations for pregnancy among diabetic women, or do you find some other reasons that are more common?

DR. LOIS: Personally, I think that diabetic women are overachievers because diabetes only happens to highly motivated, talented people! Your stories above are true, however.

JUNE AND BARBARA: Dr. Janet Mitchell, the director of a high-risk pregnancy unit at Beth Israel hospital in Boston, has noticed that husbands tend to be more unsettled than their wives by hazardous pregnancies—"The mother puts the baby first, but he puts the mother first." Have you noticed this, too? If so, how do you think it affects the dynamics of the pregnancy?

DR. LOIS: Yes, husbands do have trouble with a rocky course in pregnancy. They think it is their role to protect and care for their wives, and they feel impotent when the wife becomes sick or the baby is in jeopardy. It is also harder to have your beloved sick than to be sick yourself. These two emotions potentiate each other and can cause extreme anxiety.

One way to help alleviate the problem is to give the husband tasks and responsibilities, such as mixing and administering glucagon, if necessary, or waking up at 3 A.M. to help the wife do a middle-of-the-night blood-sugar check. During labor, husbands are also useful to perform the blood-sugar checks while the woman is busy doing her Lamaze breathing.

JUNE AND BARBARA: The *New York Times* article on chronically ill women who decide to have children also pointed out that "other family members, especially children, are marked when a sick woman embarks on motherhood. Sometimes a mother is bedridden or limited in her physical activities. There may be tension in the house, which adults often try to hide. Always, children are asked to do more, tolerate more, understand more than those with healthy mothers."

Assuming that this is so, do you have any suggestions as to how the tensions can be diminished?

DR. LOIS: Yes. Family therapy is needed for even the best-adjusted families. Often, there are many painful issues that are not discussed. Group therapy facilitates the verbalization of anger, pain, and rejection. A child may feel unloved because Mommy eats first. The issue is a feeling of a lack of love, not an issue of the timing of dinner. Perhaps in other subconscious ways the mother has ignored the child's needs, a situation that would be easy to remedy if only she were aware of it.

The best way to have a child accept the mother's diabetes is to include the child on all blood-sugar checks and injections.

Whenever my kids fell and skinned a knee, instead of a bandage we would run for a blood-sugar check. After all, it was a free way to check the sugar, since they were bleeding anyway. My kids also know how to help me help myself whenever I am low. I need all the help I can get at those times. Let me share with you a letter from a patient of mine:

Luke saved the day for me shortly after Andrew was born. My husband was working nights at the time, and Luke (who had just turned four) woke up and came into my bed and found me barely conscious. My blood sugar was so low I couldn't talk to tell him what I needed. Luke got on the phone and dialed "0," told the operator I was sick and needed an ambulance. Thank God I taught him our address, which he gave to the operator. The operator kept him on the phone until the ambulance and police arrived and he let them in. Luke never panicked or cried, and stayed with me and the baby watching over us to make sure they didn't do anything wrong. He even showed them where I kept my meter and my husband's work number so he could come home. I was so proud—so happy I had talked to him about what to do in case of an emergency. For a while after that he was always watching what I ate; he was afraid of it happening again.

The only bad part of that experience was I couldn't tell them where the glucagon was, so they gave me tons of sugar in orange juice. When I was finally on my feet and tested my blood, it read "high" on my meter. But I was alive.

JUNE AND BARBARA: Some couples fear pregnancy for a very realistic reason: they're afraid they won't be able to afford it. Concerning the expense of a diabetic woman's pregnancy, we remember the story in our *The Diabetic's Book* about a doctor who always calls in the bride's and the groom's parents. He asks, "Do you want to be grandparents? Okay, then, are you willing to help out with the medical expenses of the pregnancy?" The future grandparents always say yes, the doctor reported, and he added with a smile, "I always hold them to their word."

Amy, a diabetic friend of ours, had expenses in 1986 that were doubtless much higher than most because of the relatively expensive hospital she went to and because of the thoroughness of the monitoring of the unborn child. She had two amniocenteses at $675 each, four ultrasounds at $275 each, two fetal echo checks at $300 each, and eight fetal nonstress tests at about $75 each.

All this comes to a tidy $3,650. Also, the baby was in intensive care in the neonatal unit of the hospital for the first one or two days.

What is your assessment of the cost factor?

**DR. LOIS:** The economics of a pregnancy complicated by diabetes have actually improved. Before home blood-glucose monitoring, a woman would be hospitalized for over half her pregnancy, so the usual hospital bill in 1980 was around $40,000. In 1995 this same bill would be closer to $120,000. But now the cost of home monitoring of glucose (six tests daily for nine months) and professional care is closer to $4,000.

Now the major expense is fetal monitoring and testing. There is good news on the horizon, however, for as better tests become available the present protocols for multiple serial tests may become obsolete. These newer tests of fetal blood-vessel-flow parameters must be verified to correctly predict the fetus at risk before they become a part of clinical care. In the meantime, repetitive serial fetal monitoring is the only available tool we have to assure the obstetrician that the unborn child is safe inside.

**JUNE AND BARBARA:** When our friend Amy was thinking about getting pregnant, one of her biggest worries was her age. At thirty-five, she knew the biological time clock might have ticked too long. Her concern was whether there is an age cutoff time at which it becomes inordinately risky for a diabetic woman to become pregnant.

**DR. LOIS:** No, there isn't. But after the age of thirty-five *any* woman should have a test to ensure that mongolism does not occur. This is a test of the baby's chromosomes to see whether they are normal. All women over the age of thirty-five have a one-in-forty chance of having a genetically defective child. Whether or not they have diabetes does not increase this risk. Nor does it decrease the risk; diabetic women still suffer the ailments of normal women.

No matter how old a diabetic woman is, she should complete the following four steps before conception:

1. Consultation with an ophthalmologist to assure that eye status is stable
2. Normal blood-pressure test and normal twenty-four-hour urine test for kidney function
3. Normal gynecological examination
4. Normal glycosylated-hemoglobin level

An okay on all of the above points gives permission to become pregnant.

JUNE AND BARBARA: We would imagine that diabetes care differs somewhat while a woman is carrying her baby. What changes does a woman have to make in her self-therapy?

DR. LOIS: She has to maintain the same good care as always, only more so. Pregnancy means an intensification of the self-care program. The goal is to maintain constant normal blood sugars. By normal I mean premeal blood sugars of 60 to 90 mg/dl and one-hour postmeal blood sugars of less than 140 mg/dl. The rule is that the better the mother's blood-sugar level, the better the baby. The only way to keep such strict control of blood-sugar levels is to check the level on a meter between five and ten times a day.

The total program consists of blood-sugar monitoring

combined with at least three daily insulin injections and rigid meal planning (three meals and four snacks daily). With this kind of commitment to self-care, a diabetic woman can have a perfectly normal, healthy baby. Without it, the outcome of pregnancy can be much less than ideal. This is well verified by the fact that before 1922, when insulin became commercially available, no infant of a diabetic mother survived. Even after insulin came on the scene, up to 50 percent of pregnancies terminated in stillbirth. Today, a diabetic woman has the same chance of delivering a normal, healthy baby as a nondiabetic woman.

For a detailed view of diabetes management during a pregnancy, please consult the supplement at the end of the book.

JUNE AND BARBARA: One of our questioners had heard a diabetic woman must stay in bed during the last two months of pregnancy. Is this true?

DR. LOIS: No. Diabetic women do not need to stay in bed. Bed rest is the preferred treatment for high blood pressure, preeclampsia (a toxic syndrome of pregnancy), and premature dilation of the cervix or premature labor. If a diabetic woman needs to stay in bed it is because she has one of these problems, *not* because of the diabetes itself.

JUNE AND BARBARA: Many people have made the observation that diabetic women seem to have fat babies. Is this always the case?

DR. LOIS: This is known as the "Big Bad Baby" syndrome and is totally preventable. In the past, many diabetic women did give birth to babies weighing more than twelve pounds. The dynamics of this phenomenon are simple.

At about the twenty-sixth week of pregnancy, the infant has a fully formed pancreas that is capable of secreting its own insulin. If the mother has abnormally high blood-glucose levels, the sugar crosses the placenta to the baby. The baby will work to lower the blood sugar by producing extra insulin in its pancreas, which causes the baby to grow bigger. Just as a person becomes fat by eating too much, the developing baby becomes fat when too much sugar is transported into its circulation.

On the other hand, if the blood-glucose level of the mother is normal, then the baby will not become "big and bad." All you have to do to cure the Big Bad Baby syndrome is to absolutely normalize blood-glucose levels during pregnancy.

JUNE AND BARBARA: Another important question asked repeatedly is whether a diabetic woman has to have a cesarean instead of a normal delivery.

DR. LOIS: No. A cesarean delivery is only indicated in specific cases. The indications of a c-section are:

1. Too large a baby to delivery vaginally
2. Malpresentation (breech)
3. Uterine pathology
4. Dysfunctional labor
5. Repeat c-section

Problems two through five can happen to any woman, but problem one is usually a problem associated with diabetes. Good glucose control during pregnancy can help prevent the baby from becoming too fat. Thus, a woman can do something to decrease her chances of a c-section.

Previously, doctors delivered women with diabetes before the due date, when it was too early for vaginal delivery. Now, with improved glucose control and up-to-date fetal monitoring, the pregnancy can progress to the due date, and successful vaginal delivery is thus more likely.

JUNE AND BARBARA: How about the other type of pregnancy with diabetes, when the woman develops diabetes in the middle of her term, though she wasn't diabetic before that?

DR. LOIS: In my fifteen years of experience providing medical care to more than five hundred pregnant women with diabetes, more than half of these women were diagnosed with having gestational diabetes. In fact, there are around five hundred thousand cases of this type of pregnancy in the United States every year. Fortunately, the mother's diabetes is largely a temporary condition and disappears when she gives birth, but she does have a high risk (between 25 and 60 percent) of developing permanent diabetes later in life.

The baby does not know what type of diabetes the mother has. Therefore, it is just as important to maintain normal blood sugars during a pregnancy complicated by gestational diabetes to assure a normal, healthy infant as it is with a Type I pregnancy. In gestational diabetes the mother must have an appropriate diet and an exercise plan just as with Type I mothers, but not all gestational diabetics need insulin injections. For an overview of caring for yourself during a gestational pregnancy, please consult the supplement at the end of the book.

JUNE AND BARBARA: One diabetic woman who had her baby when she was in her thirties looked aghast when she was asked if she were going to have another. "Not on your life!" was her unequivocal reply. Although hers was not a complicated pregnancy and things went very smoothly, she couldn't take the thought of all those low blood sugars and all the constant monitoring. She was so tired of coping with her physiology that she didn't even want to nurse. It wasn't that she regretted in the slightest having her baby—he is the greatest joy of her and her husband's lives. But she had not the slightest desire to do it again. Her attitude was rather like the Japanese saying about climbing Mount Fuji: "He who doesn't do it once is a big fool. He who does it twice is a bigger fool."

Of course, this woman made these negative statements only a couple of months after the birth, and she may change her mind later. But do you generally find that once is enough for most diabetic women?

DR. LOIS: Actually, I have found that most women have a letdown after the baby is born. They find that they are no longer special and no longer need extra attention; they not involved in a miracle anymore. Somehow, being a nonpregnant diabetic woman does not hold the same glamour and require the same degree of care that a pregnant, high-risk diabetic woman has. During the ten years of our pregnancy and diabetes program in New York, three of my patients have had three children each, and twenty-two have had two. The remaining ninety-five have had only one baby each.

JUNE AND BARBARA: You mentioned the letdown after the baby is born. One woman—diabetic since the age of nine—who had had two successful pregnancies wrote to us hoping that in this new edition you would address postpartum "adjustment," as she prefers to call it. She said that as difficult and intensive as her pregnancies were, they were nothing compared to what she went through the first few months following delivery. "Both times I was an absolute mess. Aside from all the hormonal adjustments, my blood sugars tended to fluctuate anywhere between 30 and 300 in a matter of hours. This took a tremendous toll on me emotionally. I felt totally out of control. I tried to explain to my family that this was a very difficult time for me, but nobody in my family—not even my husband or mother—seemed to understand or accept what I was going through. I am willing to bet that I am not the only diabetic woman to experience this."

DR. LOIS: She wins her bet! Every woman experiences similar symptoms after her baby is born. When the placenta—a busy, around-the-clock "hormone factory"—is delivered, there is a sudden precipitous drop in the new mother's hormone levels. This produces a "hormone withdrawal." It is as though a pregnant woman becomes addicted to the high levels of hormones and then is expected to quit her addiction cold turkey at the moment of the birth.

This sudden hormone withdrawal causes:

**1. Severe mood swings and depression.**

**2. A precipitous drop in insulin requirement.**
   In addition, if a woman breast-feeds, her insulin requirement changes based on when and how much milk the baby nurses. All women find the postpartum period to be an emotional roller coaster, but diabetic women are also blessed with a sugar roller coaster. The challenge is to discover the right doses of insulin you need

during this period. To do this, you must consult the best and most experienced diabetes health-care people available. You can help them in the discovery process by charting all the foods you consume, the times of nursing, your emotional highs and lows, and your sleep patterns. On top of that you should do six to ten blood sugar tests a day: before and after each meal, before and after each nursing session, after an emotional high or low, etc., and record in detail the results of these tests.

The Bible talks about the need to pamper a woman after she gives birth. She is sent away from the community (especially from her husband and mother!) to be cared for by "gentle women," only to return when she is fully recovered and has regained a sense of control. So you see, the wise scholars of the past knew about post-partum blues. We just need to reinstitute their solutions.

JUNE AND BARBARA: We'd like to know if there is any optimal number of children a diabetic woman should have. Do the risks increase with each pregnancy?

DR. LOIS: Diabetic women have the same chances as nondiabetic women. If a woman has a c-section for the first child, she will usually have c-sections for the rest of her children. Four are quite enough of that!

Also, in each subsequent gestational diabetic pregnancy the gestational diabetes gets worse.

JUNE AND BARBARA: As an only child herself, Barbara feels they're not as bad as they're portrayed in legend and song. But do you find that many diabetic women do not like the idea of bringing up a spoiled, self-centered, lonely only child? And if so, do they sometimes opt for adoption after the first pregnancy?

DR. LOIS: Sometimes, yes. Many of my patients have chosen to devote nine months of their lives to making a healthy baby, and they then adopt a second child to complete their family rather than stealing time from the first child to devote another nine months to intense self-care.

JUNE AND BARBARA: Now there's a Brave New World alternative to adoption: fertilizing in vitro with the husband's sperm and the wife's egg and using a surrogate mother to carry the baby. The husband of a woman who had such an extremely difficult first pregnancy that her tubes had been tied asked us about the possibility of having a second child using a surrogate. Actually they were convinced that was what they wanted to do. The problem was that her endocrinologist wanted her to have a normal $A_{1C}$ before the egg was taken so that there would be no danger of its being damaged by high blood sugars. A normal $A_{1C}$ is extremely difficult for her to obtain because she has potential kidney problems, can eat very little protein, and is pretty much restricted to carbohydrates, which, of course, are what raise blood sugar. Have you heard of many diabetic women using surrogates? If so, how did they work out?

DR. LOIS: If this couple goes for a baby by surrogate, then during the stimulation cycle (the menstrual cycle in which hormones are given to the woman to stimulate the growth of many eggs) the blood-glucose levels should be optimal. Because the estrogen levels rise very high during a stimulation cycle to obtain eggs, the easiest plan would be to wear an insulin pump. Then the basal rate of insulin can be adjusted upward as the hormones rise and need more insulin. Of course, in order to adjust the pump, at least eight blood-glucose levels need to be made daily—premeal and postmeal, at bedtime, and at 3 A.M.

Surrogates are now more common, but since this type of procedure is a private, delicate issue, most women do not share their experiences. This is why the true number of diabetic women using surrogates is unknown.

JUNE AND BARBARA: The woman we mentioned who felt once was enough said that her husband is even more adamant than she—he absolutely refuses to go through it all again. Donna Jornsay, the diabetic woman who was quoted in the *New York Times* article "Having Children Despite Illness," made it sound as though her husband might echo those sentiments. She said he stopped sleeping during her ninth month of pregnancy because he was so afraid she would go into coma. The idea was so terrifying to him that he would wake her up as many as twenty times a night to make sure she was all right. She felt he was relieved when she was hospitalized because it was no longer his responsibility to keep her alive. Do you find this usual among husbands of diabetic women?

DR. LOIS: Yes, if the husband does not know what to do to prevent the problem from occurring or to treat the problem if it does happen. Blood-glucose levels can be terrifying, but most of the time the insulin and/or the food pattern can be corrected to prevent unconsciousness due to extreme hypoglycemia.

JUNE AND BARBARA: When Amy became pregnant, her doctor wanted her to keep her blood sugar between 80 and 120. This meant that, working this close to the line, she had to endure a number of rather dramatic hypoglycemic incidents. Once she almost passed out at work. Is extremely low blood sugar harmful for the baby?

DR. LOIS: Transient hypoglycemia does not harm the unborn child. However, *hyper*glycemia (any blood sugar greater than 140) may harm fetus; thus, for the sake of the fetus, it's worth running the risk of hypoglycemia to ensure that hyperglycemia does not happen.

Hypoglycemia is not, of course, pleasant for mothers-to-be and their anxious husbands, and there is no reason to put up with hypoglycemia if a change in insulin dose, diet, or exercise can fix the problem without causing hyperglycemia. Perhaps decreasing the dose of insulin per injection and increasing the number of injections will do the trick; perhaps adding between-meal snacks or changing to pump therapy will smooth out the glucose levels.

An important thing to remember is that the greatest risk to the fetus is a *swift change* in blood glucose. For instance, if a pregnant woman has blood sugar low enough to make her unconscious or unable to eat, her husband may panic and call an ambulance. The medics are trained to give large intravenous doses of sugar to any unconscious diabetic person, and blood glucose could thus go from 20 to 600 in minutes. While the level of 20 is probably not bothering the fetus, the swift change in glucose to severely hyperglycemic levels does harm the fetus.

Therefore, husbands should be trained in how to inject glucagon, just in case. The husband can be instructed to give half the dose to his wife, wait ten minutes, and then give the other half, if necessary. This two-dose treatment minimizes the chance of overdosing initially. Once the woman is "with it," usually within fifteen minutes, she can check her blood sugar and eat food to induce the hypoglycemia to gently come back into the normal ranges.

**JUNE AND BARBARA:** What do you recommend for treating hypoglycemia for your pregnant women?

**DR. LOIS:** I recommend eight ounces of milk for a blood sugar documented to be less than 70 and associated with hypoglycemia symptoms. (A 60 may be normal if it's *stable*, but it may have been caught only while a woman was on her way down to zero.) Recheck the blood sugar in fifteen minutes and drink another glass of milk if necessary. Recheck again in fifteen minutes, and if the level is less than 70 drink a third glass of milk and eat a slice of bread. For minor hypoglycemia, most women do not require the third glass of milk.

If a woman is unresponsive or is unable to eat, then glucagon must be subcutaneously injected.

**JUNE AND BARBARA:** Since the recommended blood-sugar levels for a pregnant diabetic woman are lower than for the general diabetic population, could you give us some guidelines?

**DR. LOIS:** Yes. They are:

Prebreakfast (fasting) goal: 55–70 mg/dl
Prelunch goal: 55–70 mg/dl
One hour after each meal: below 140 mg/dl
Average blood sugar of all the premeals and all the postmeals (six per day) should be 80–85 mg/dl.

**JUNE AND BARBARA:** Since these numbers differ from the standard normal range, should a pregnant woman's hemoglobin $A_{1C}$ (the every-three-months monitor of blood glucose levels) be different, too?

DR. LOIS: Yes, because pregnancy demands that the mean blood glucose be lower than for nonpregnant persons. Therefore, the "normal range" for most lab glycosylated-hemoglobin levels cannot be used to determine whether a pregnant woman is in good control. The ideal lab would be one that also has pregnancy norms. (For more details on this, see the Type I Pregnancy Supplement.)

JUNE AND BARBARA: Some women use an insulin-infusion pump during pregnancy. Is this recommended?

DR. LOIS: Not necessarily. Pumps create special problems during pregnancy. Since there are no subcutaneous stores of insulin when a woman is on a pump, if the needle slips for more than four hours she can go into ketoacidosis. In addition, because of the change in skin sweat and temperature, it is easier to develop an infection at the needle site. Infection necessitates antibiotics and usually causes the blood glucose to rise, two situations that are definitely not wanted during pregnancy.

It is therefore not recommended that a woman be on a pump during pregnancy, but it is certainly worse to be in poor glucose control during pregnancy. Pregnancy is a special time during which permission is automatically granted to eat special foods, eat when no one else eats, test blood sugars frequently, sleep sufficiently, and so on. It is not a selfish act to spend time caring for yourself, for you are also caring for your unborn child.

Thus, it is somehow easier to take the time for three injections and five to seven blood-glucose tests a day. The nonpregnant diabetic does not have this luxury in real life; the pregnant woman needs all the help she can get to make diabetes self-care easier. Therefore, I would never prescribe a pump for her. She can do equally as well on multiple injections. However, for the woman who is *planning* a pregnancy, I would prescribe the pump to help her get her act in order before pregnancy. Then when she gets pregnant she can stay on the pump, but must be fastidious about her needle site.

JUNE AND BARBARA: We know a diabetic woman who's had diabetes for about twenty-six years who vomited throughout her entire pregnancy. She did have some kidney problems during the pregnancy. What would be the reason for the vomiting? Does it happen frequently and is there a way to prevent it?

DR. LOIS: The word for severe vomiting during pregnancy is *hyperemesis gravidarum*. The general philosophy is that it is a result of the combination of the hormones of pregnancy and an element of psychological maladjustment to the pregnancy. However, high hormone levels of twins commonly cause severe morning sickness, even when a woman is well adjusted to the pregnancy. Eating frequent small, bland meals helps. Also, hypoglycemic reaction can make the nausea worse. Thus, the treatment plan should include small doses of Regular insulin before very small meals (six per day). In addition, kidney failure can cause nausea all by itself; thus pregnancy plus kidney problems can mean nausea without implicating a psychological component.

JUNE AND BARBARA: Is it okay for a diabetic woman to breast-feed her baby, and, if so, are there any special precautions she should take?

DR. LOIS: I firmly believe that if a woman with diabetes keeps her blood-glucose levels normal before and throughout pregnancy, she can have a normal infant. Why, then, should there be any reason not to breast-feed?

Before I began to advocate breast-feeding for my diabetic women patients, however, I wanted to be sure that it would be best for the baby. So we set up an experiment to look at the relationship of maternal blood glucose and insulin to milk glucose and insulin. We learned that the higher the mother's blood sugar, the sweeter the milk. In addition, insulin comes into the milk freely. We do not know the implications for the baby of drinking sugar-laden milk with regard to taste and preference and/or subsequent obesity and eating disorders. We do know that the insulin will not hurt the infant. (If insulin could be put into a glass of milk to make it work, none of us would inject it!) Therefore, the rule of thumb for assuring the most normal nutrition for the baby is that women should keep themselves in the best possible control.

We have learned that women must adjust their insulin dosages frequently while they are breast-feeding, because as the baby grows more sugar is siphoned to it. Usually, the increased food intake during the day compensates for this, but when the baby eats at 11 P.M. and 3 A.M., the next result is that the bedtime insulins must be cut way back. In fact, many women skip the bedtime dose of NPH insulin altogether. The other option is to overeat before bed to prevent a hypoglycemic reaction. However, most postpartum women are desperate to lose weight, and forcing themselves to eat at bedtime is therefore depressing.

JUNE AND BARBARA: One diabetic mother wrote of a worry that must be common to all diabetic mothers of small children:

One major problem I encountered as a diabetic mother was the possibility of having a severe insulin reaction when I was home alone with my baby and young children. I had no relatives living nearby, and for a while no close neighbors, as we lived in the country.

To have someone check on me meant letting someone know where I was at all times. If they phoned while I was changing a diaper, out in the garden, or in town on errands, it would be a false alarm. If we arranged a preset time to call, what about all the hours in between when an insulin reaction could occur? My ultimate solution was to keep my blood sugars high at all times—this was in the days before home blood-sugar monitors. My husband was away a fair amount of the time on overnight business trips, which didn't help, either. My doctors told me I was damaging my health, but no doctor ever came up with a better solution.

DR. LOIS: As she mentioned in passing, the blood-glucose monitoring that is now possible diminishes the problem. It doesn't mean, however, that low blood-sugar incidents can't happen to a diabetic mother.

One way she can avoid these is by realizing the times of potential hypoglycemia danger, based on when her insulin peaks and will drive down her blood sugar. For example, if she is on a program of NPH and regular insulin, blood-sugar tests *must* be performed two and a half hours after Regular is injected and eight hours after NPH is injected. *Any* blood sugar less than 100 should be treated with milk until the blood sugar is greater than 100.

JUNE AND BARBARA: Since youth is so revered in this country, many diabetic (and nondiabetic!) women find moving into the *troisième âge* a depressing stage in life.

We hope to be able to prove to you that it ain't necessarily so.

## Le Troisième Age

According to Robert Browning, this is the "best is yet to be" time. Poetic though his phrase may be, you may consider it unrealistic or even stupid. But it can be true. Your family responsibilities are diminished, and you can finally begin to think of yourself—your health, your interests, your career goals—and even, at least occasionally, put them first. In a sense you are truly free to be the real you—and think of the reduction in stress that can entail if you've been role-playing to please others for as long as you can remember. As one woman remarked during a heated prochoice/right-to-life discussion about when life begins, "With all due respect, I think life begins when the children leave home and the dog dies." *Le troisième âge* can be the beginning of your life, your real life, the life in which you can amaze everyone—including yourself—at what you can achieve and what excitement you can stir up. To quote scholar and mystery writer Dorothy L. Sayers, "Time and trouble will tame an advanced young woman, but an advanced old woman is uncontrollable by any earthly force."

Moving into *le troisième âge* also is a proverbial wake-up call. If you're ever going to seize the day, you have to grab it now. Then, just in case you pressed the snooze button and turned over to doze a little longer, along came diabetes buzzing loudly to once and for all blast you out of your somnolence. You now have two clear signals that you are mortal, that your time is not infinite. Rather than being a dismal realization, it can be a very good thing for you. According to author, educator, and love guru Leo Buscaglia, the happiest people he knows are those who have a sense of their own mortality. They are the ones who realize how precious every remaining day is, so they fill each one with all the joy and satisfying accomplishment it can hold.

The newspapers are full of stories of day-seizing woman in their fifties and sixties and even beyond making dramatic career changes. At fifty-seven Helen Johnson of Greendale, Wisconsin, went back to school and became a teacher; then at seventy-seven she learned to drive a truck—a twelve-ton rig! Shortly thereafter, she made the truck run from her home to El Salvador! Mavis Lindgren started an exercise program to improve her health at age sixty-two. One thing led to another until, seven years later, she ran her first marathon. Soon thereafter she began gathering up world marathon records in her age class. The last report we heard of Mavis was that she was celebrating her eighty-eighth birthday by running in The World's Largest Marathon in London. Harriet Doerr started college in 1927 and dropped out in her sophomore year to get married. After her children and grandchildren grew up, she returned to finish college and started trying her hand at fiction writing. Her first novel, the best-selling *Stones for Ibarra*, was published when she was seventy-three. She's still at it with another best-seller, *Consider This, Señora*.

You may say, but these women didn't have diabetes. Yet if you thumb through a few issues of *Diabetes Forecast*, you'll find equally inspiring stories of *troisième âge* diabetic women. June detests it when Barbara uses her as a living, go-thou-and-do-likewise example and even forbids her to do so, but when it's appropriate, Barbara does it anyway. So here goes. In the first edition of this book it was reported that in the third age, after retiring at age sixty-two from her thirty-five-year career as a librarian, she became happier and more productive (working nine-to-ten-hour days and seven-day weeks when necessary) than ever before—starting a business and writing more, engaging in more sports activities. Nine years later, it still holds true. In 1990 she retired from one business, the SugarFree Center, and quickly joined in the starting of another, Prana Publications. She has subsequently been a participant in the writing of four more books and a new semiannual newsletter, *The Diabetic Reader*. In 1992 to celebrate her twenty-fifth diabetes anniversary—still without complications—she went on what they call in Germany a *Wanderjahr* (year of travel). During this year she went on trips to Florence, Paris, Switzerland, Montana, Wisconsin, New York, Hong Kong, and Bali, plus brief forays to San Francisco and Santa Barbara. (She's already looking forward to doing more of the same on her fiftieth diabetes anniversary, and, of course Barbara will be goading her on, as usual.) She's given up skiing, mainly because of fear of the Demon Snowboarder, but, despite a broken arm from a skid and fall from biking over a rain-slicked railroad track, she still dreams of getting back on her mountain bike again. (It may never happen, but you gotta have dreams—as well as heart.) She remains an enthusiastic walker despite foot surgery for a couple of neuromas. She is looking forward to *never* retiring.

Many diabetic women her age are doing as much as this—or more. But, unfortunately, many others in the *troisième âge* are not. We see women every day who seem to have given up on life and on themselves and who use their age and their diabetes as their excuse.

We've also noticed that a sadly large number of third-age women approach everything new with negative expectations. This is particularly true when it comes to learning how to use a blood-sugar meter. These meters are easier than ever to use, having been carefully designed so that a person of normal intelligence and dexterity can operate them with no difficulty. Yet these women approach the meters with fear and trembling, and they often come right out and say, "This is too much for me" or "I just can't handle mechanical things." Even if they don't say it, it's written all over their faces. And you know what? It turns out that these women *can't* work the meters. They can have lesson after lesson and explanation after explanation, and they still don't get it. Why? *Because they're certain they're not going to.* That negative certainty is like a lead shield dropping down and blocking all learning.

One of the participants in the Iron Man triathlon (participants swim 2.4 miles, bicycle 112 miles, and run 26 miles—all in one day!) recently said that the moment you start thinking you can't do it, it's all over. The negative thoughts will beat you every time. On the other hand, if you say over and over, like the little engine that could, "I think I can! I think I can!" then the battle's more than half won.

The other half of the battle involves taking the time to learn to do it right. In his book *The Road Less Traveled*, M. Scott Peck writes, "I and anyone who is not mentally defective can solve any problem if we are willing to take the time. . . . Many people simply do not take the time to solve problems."

Sitting down calmly and taking the time to really understand how to use a meter or any other product or piece of equipment associated with your diabetes care will pay tremendous dividends, and not just in improved diabetes control. A more important dividend is that you will learn, as Dr. Peck believes, that most of life's mechanical, intellectual, social, and spiritual problems are solvable if you are just willing both to take the time and to make the necessary changes.

*Question:* How many psychologists does it take to change a lightbulb?

*Answer:* Only one, but it can take a very long time, and the lightbulb has to really *want* to change.

It's even harder to change a person than a lightbulb—especially if that person has become somewhat set in her ways over the years. When you come right down to it, people can't be changed. They have to change themselves. But change they must, because changing is the key to survival and happiness.

This is particularly true for diabetic people, who, especially at first, have to make a huge number of changes. But there are rewards for your efforts: the reward of improved health and appearance and, best of all, the reward of becoming a person who is capable of making changes in all areas of life—in other words, a winner.

This resiliency is also a hallmark of youth. A *première âge* person who cannot make changes is an old person, but a person in the *troisième âge* who can make changes is young, whatever her birth certificate may say. So if you get your diabetes later in life, as many Type II diabetics do, you can regard it and the changes it causes you to make as rejuvenating forces.

"Great," you may say, "I have this diabetes and I need to make changes, and I know that if I do it will make a lot of big, positive differences in my life. But how do I *motivate* myself to make these changes?"

Motivation. Aye, there's the rub. It would be hard to count the number of sessions we've attended at diabetes conferences that deal with motivation and how diabetes health professionals can motivate their patients to start doing all the things they need to do.

After a great deal of thought in the matter, we've come to this conclusion:

## DOWN WITH MOTIVATION!

We hear it almost every day: "(Heavy sigh) I just can't get myself motivated to . . . (lose weight, exercise every day, start testing my blood sugar, etc.)."

We have news for you. Motivation is not going to strike you like lightning. And motivation is not something that someone else—nurse, doctor, family member, friend—can bestow or force upon you. The whole idea of motivation is a trap. Just get in there and take the first step to lose weight, exercise, test your blood sugar, or whatever. Do it *without* motivation. And then, guess what? After you start actually doing whatever it is, *that's* when motivation comes and makes it easier for you to keep on doing it. There was one overweight woman whom we were encouraging to start exercising. We made a deal with her: she was to walk around the block every day for a week and then call and tell us how it felt.

She didn't want to, and she groaned a lot, but she agreed to do it. A week later she called and admitted that while she had hated doing it the first time, it had gotten a tiny bit better every day, until by the end of the week it wasn't bad at all. Since then she's gradually increased her daily walk to two miles, and she has her husband out walking with her. Now they're so motivated to keep it up that they seldom miss a day.

Motivation is like happiness—it's a by-product. When you're actively engaged in Doing Something, motivation sneaks up and zaps you when you least expect it. As Harvard psychologist Jerome Bruner says, "You're more likely to act yourself into feeling than feel yourself into action." So act! Read what Dr. Lois tells you to do as a Type II diabetic, then leap up and do it!

JUNE AND BARBARA: Diana Guthrie, an eminent diabetes nurse-educator at the Kansas Regional Medical Center in Wichita, once told us that the diabetics who most often come into the hospital with serious problems are Type II's who have been ignoring their conditions. What advice do you have for these people, and what recommendations can you give for their preventive care?

DR. LOIS: High blood glucose is associated with an increased risk of heart disease and stroke. In fact, even people with borderline glucose intolerance (high blood sugars but not high enough to meet the definition of diabetes) have an increased risk. Therefore, as healthcare professionals interested in preventive medicine, we should lower the blood-glucose level back down toward normal.

There are several risk factors that potentiate the risk of heart attack and stroke:

1.  Hyperglycemia
2.  Hypertension
3.  Smoking
4.  Sedentary lifestyle
5.  Being male
6.  Aging
7.  High uric acid (gout)

Although obesity carries with it a higher risk of sedentary life, high blood glucose, and diabetes, a fat person who has normal blood pressure and normal blood sugar and who leads an active life is not at risk. Thus, obesity is not a risk factor all by itself. Therefore, although I push diet as the mainstay of therapy for Type II diabetic women, I would not be a good physician if I gave up on the patient if she could not lose weight. I would try to bring the blood-glucose level down with pills and/or insulin if necessary and vigorously treat the blood pressure, start the patient on an exercise program, treat the gout (hyperuricemia), and be vehement about not smoking.

I ran the diabetes clinic for seven years at the New York Hospital. Of the 1,000 patients who registered in that clinic during that time, 85 percent were obese, Type II diabetic women. I learned a lot from these women. Basically, they educated me on how to understand them.

Many of these women had had a lifelong problem with obesity. How could I reverse a lifetime of poor eating habits in one clinic visit? Clearly, a busy physician is not the right person to implement behavior modification. But I could direct the patient to a better support system—a dietitian who would translate my diet prescription into a meal plan, a diabetes educator to teach foot care and sick-day rules and reinforce blood-glucose testing techniques, an exercise program exclusively for overweight women so they could feel comfortable wearing leotards, and a group therapy directed toward the chronic eating disorder. My role as the physician then became the coordinator and monitor of success. If my plan failed, then I could shift gears and begin again.

Although many of my patients did not lose weight, I improved the average glycosylated hemoglobin in our clinic by two percentage points.

I guess that I have only one standard of care. Since Type II diabetic women are older, I view each Type II woman as though she were my mother. "If this were my mother," I found myself saying, "then I would make sure that her blood-glucose levels were below the levels of risk for heart attack and stroke." The safe zone appears to be a fasting blood glucose of below 110 mg/dl and postprandial levels below 165 mg/dl. If I cannot help a patient to achieve this degree of control, I send her to a doctor who may have a different approach, one that is more effective for this patient, for I am not helping her as long as her glucose levels are in the risk zone.

Blood-glucose self-monitoring is a beautiful way to assess dietary management. If the meal plan is perfect, the postmeal glucose level should be below 165 mg/dl. If a patient measures her blood glucose one hour after the meal and finds her blood glucose to be above 165 mg/dl, we can then discuss what foods in that meal she did not tolerate. Was it the ketchup, because I forgot to teach her that ketchup has sugar? Was it the soup with hidden items that are not easily accounted for? Talking about the blood glucose takes the emphasis off the scale. Many of my patients would rather skip a visit than step on a scale. So I do not weigh my patients. Why should I, if obesity alone is not harmful?

JUNE AND BARBARA: You mentioned bringing down blood-glucose levels of Type II women with pills that lower blood sugar if these women can't get into control with diet. Could you explain the use of these pills? Many people have the false impression that these are insulin pills. When June was diagnosed as having diabetes at the age of forty-five, she was considered a Type II and was allowed to try three of the pills—Orinase, Tolinase, and Diabinese—but they did not lower her blood sugar enough to prevent her from having to go onto insulin.

DR. LOIS: Those three pills belong to the sulfonylurea family of drugs. The second generation of sulfonylurea compounds has since been introduced in this country in the form of glipizide and glyburide. These two agents do not cause salt and water retention, as Diabinese did, and they can be given in very small doses. The small dose is an advantage because the side effect of abnormal heart rhythm is also less. These new agents can be given in one-hundredth of the dose of the first-generation pills. It is easy to outeat these pills, however, and therefore putting a patient on such a pill does not give her permission to stop her diet.

There is one new drug on the market called metformin with the brand name Glucophage. It has been available in the rest of the world for fifteen years. It is a "sister" to a pill available about twenty years ago called phenformin, which was a wonderful treatment for Type II's, but it was taken off the market because there was a very small risk of side effects. The side effect they were worried about was lactic acidosis. (A build up of lactate in the bloodstream which, in high levels, makes the bloodstream acidic.) Metformin does not cause this problem, except if it is abused. And thus we welcome back this beneficent family of pills.

Metformin lowers the sugar by preventing sugar release from the liver (the major cause of the high morning blood sugars) and improves the sugar usage by muscle. It does not cause the pancreas to secrete more insulin. This makes it especially useful for the treatment of Type II's. Type II's paradoxically make too much insulin, and these large quantities of circulating insulin actually limit the insulin's potency by creating a resistance to itself. That is why a treatment that lowers blood sugar without raising the insulin level even higher is ideal.

There is also another new class of oral agents on the horizon. "Starch blockers," or acarbose, is an alpha glucosidase inhibitor. This means that it blocks the enzyme that helps us absorb starches. Therefore, acarbose is useful for the management of Type II's who have carbohydrate (starch) intolerance. The starch then passes from the stomach through the small intestine untouched and reaches the large bowel where all the bacteria live. The bacteria act on the starch and create gas. So whenever a Type II eats starch, the gas produced actually trains the person to stay away from starches rather like the way that Antabuse trains alcoholics away from alcohol by making them vomit when they imbibe.

We also have insulin sensitizers in the "warm-up" pen waiting to go to bat. These sensitizers increase the potency of insulins. Since Type II's have decreased insulin potency because their high insulin levels create resistance, this group of drugs, the "glitizones," also hold promise for Type II's.

A new idea being tried is the use of pills in combination with insulin. It has recently been reported that when bedtime NPH insulin is used to lower the following morning's wake-up blood-glucose level, the pills are effective for daytime control. The high fasting blood glucose carries with it insulin resistance, so if NPH can lower the fasting, daytime control becomes easier.

JUNE AND BARBARA: Once a Type II woman has been taught the strategy for controlling her diabetes, how can you make it work?

DR. LOIS: Honesty and trust between patient and physician are what make it work. The woman must tell me if what I have asked her to do is impossible. Then, and only then, can I tailor the plan to be right for her.

JUNE AND BARBARA: When we attended a diabetes scientific update seminar we heard a doctor speak on a study he had done on the oral hypoglycemic agent Orinase. This study was done with turkeys. The doctor explained that he had a flock of 10,000 turkeys and that he had given each turkey one Orinase tablet morning and evening for six months.

At this point in the lecture one of the physicians in the audience raised his hand and said, "Excuse me, Doctor, I don't want to interrupt your train of thought, but I have to ask you how you managed to get 10,000 turkeys to take an Orinase tablet every morning and evening."

"It was easy," replied the lecturer. "I told them that if they didn't take it, I'd put them on insulin."

But seriously, folks, this story points up the great truth that everybody has a dread of going onto insulin. That's why a typical question we get goes like this: "I have Type II diabetes, and I'm scared that my doctor will put me on insulin if my control doesn't improve. What can I do to stay off insulin? I've lost some weight on his advice, but I admit that I'm still way too heavy."

**DR. LOIS:** As many as 50 percent of all overweight Type II diabetics can control their diabetes by restricting calories and carbohydrates and eating more fiber. Not more than 40 percent of the diet should be carbohydrates. By getting your weight down by at least 20 percent you will most likely be able to control your diabetes without the use of insulin.

The reasoning behind this recommendation is that your pancreas probably *does* produce enough insulin, but your body resists the insulin. Losing weight and eating less will increase your sensitivity to insulin and improve your blood-sugar levels. The fiber in your diet will help lower your blood sugar by slowing down the absorption of glucose in the intestines. The oral hypoglycemic drugs may also help increase your sensitivity to your own insulin and prevent the need for additional injected insulin.

You can be the deciding factor in whether your doctor must prescribe pills or insulin. The goal is to normalize your blood sugar. If you can do this by following the correct diet and adding exercise to your daily program, your reward will be to stay healthy without the use of insulin injections.

JUNE AND BARBARA: The menopause is another significant life event for a woman and one about which we've received many questions, on both the physiological and the psychological aspects. Let's start with the physiology of menopause and how it can affect diabetes.

DR. LOIS: The word *menopause* comes from the Greek: *men* means "month," and *pause* means "cessation"—thus, "permanent cessation of the monthly cycle."

With this cessation of the monthly cycle, the hormones necessary to maintain this cycle deteriorate. Specifically, the female hormones estrogen and progesterone diminish. Both of these hormones counteract the action of insulin; thus, as their levels diminish in the bloodstream, insulin's action increases. The insulin requirement will drop as the menses become fewer and farther apart. If the insulin doses are not decreased, hypoglycemia results. A drop of approximately 10 to 20 percent has been noted by Type I diabetic women.

If a diabetic woman wants to take estrogen and progesterone at the time of menopause, her insulin requirement will be affected. The insulin requirement will depend on how perfectly the hormone doses match her needs. High doses of estrogen and progesterone require larger doses of insulin than low doses of estrogen and progesterone.

JUNE AND BARBARA: We've heard both pros and cons about hormonal replacement. Do you think it's a good idea?

DR. LOIS: Recently, it has been reported that estrogen plays a major role in calcium metabolism. Menopausal women are predisposed to osteoporosis (brittle bones). Better research has also shown that when estrogens are combined with progesterones to mimic the normal menstrual cycle, there is no increase in cancer. With less of a cancer scare, more physicians prescribe estrogens and progesterones to menopausal women to treat depression, hot flashes, and skin and hair changes associated with menopause—and to assure that calcium metabolism is kept normal. Most physicians will reinforce a high-calcium diet of 1,200 to 1,500 mg of calcium per day along with the hormones to keep the bones sturdy.

JUNE AND BARBARA: If a woman has a history of uterine or breast cancer, are estrogen and progesterone still considered okay?

DR. LOIS: No. Many cancers of the breast, in particular, are spread by estrogens. Although the tissue is usually tested for the estrogen receptors, it is not okay for a woman with a history of previous cancer to take estrogens because of the possibility that the cancer is sensitive to estrogens.

JUNE AND BARBARA: We read in the *New York Times* about what they called "new uses for an old class of compounds: antiestrogens." They quoted Gregory Mundy, professor of medicine at the University of Texas, who said, "Antiestrogens do all the good things estrogen does without some of the problems." Studies indicate that they block estrogen's cancer-promoting effects in tissues such as the breast and uterus. What are your feelings about these?

DR. LOIS: Although antiestrogens are still in clinical trials and will have to have a lot more extensive testing, it looks as if they could turn out to be a great alternative for women who have a personal or family history of breast cancer. They do seem to protect the bones and the heart, but they do not produce the good effects of estrogen on hot flashes and on the vaginal mucosa and the skin and hair We will also have to wait and see what may be their possible side effects.

JUNE AND BARBARA: It is very common for women— diabetic or not—to find to their distress that after the menopause or a hysterectomy they gain a lot of weight. What's the reason for this?

DR. LOIS: When a dog is spayed it becomes fat. Interesting, isn't it, since dogs don't have eating disorders! What this proves is that on one can of dog food a day, a dog that was lean and lovely before fixing can get fat and old after fixing. Therefore, to claim that a menopausal woman is getting fat because she "overeats" is a bit accusing. Actually, metabolism slows down by 25 percent after menopause, so unless the intake of food is decreased by 25 percent, the woman will gain weight.

JUNE AND BARBARA: What a rotten deal! Can nothing be done about this? Can't we rev up our metabolism in some way? For example, several authors on weight loss—including Covert Bailey, of *Fit or Fat?* fame— maintain that you can change your metabolism through a program of regular vigorous exercise so that your body will burn more calories even when you're sitting still or sleeping.

DR. LOIS: Not only can exercise metabolize glucose immediately but it also has a prolonged effect that may last up to twenty-four hours. So it is true that vigorous exercise for twenty minutes a day means more efficient fuel-burning for the rest of the day. Therefore, with exercise a woman can reverse that problem of burning 25 percent fewer calories.

JUNE AND BARBARA: The psychological problems that occur after menopause and in later life can be even more devastating than the physiological ones. Could you offer diabetic women some help and guidance in coping with these?

DR. LOIS: It's natural to grieve that you are growing older. Joints creak, a familiar flight of stairs seems to suddenly have more steps, the midline enlarges, the skin dries and wrinkles, and the hair turns gray and falls out. These physical changes certainly can be depressing for any woman, but a woman with diabetes may also perceive that she is somehow growing old *faster* than a nondiabetic friend the same age. Actually, high blood sugars do dry and scale the skin, change the vaginal secretions, and make the nails deteriorate. We used to be taught in medical school that diabetes makes people look ten years older than their chronological age. But better glucose control can slow down the aging process so that we diabetic women can suffer just like everyone else.

When a woman with diabetes goes through menopause, the emotional changes may lead to a deterioration in control. Deterioration in control increases aging, which leads to more depression. The best way for a woman to prevent this is to share the problem with a responsible diabetes health-care professional, who can take over her insulin adjustments until she is psychologically ready to take back her self-care.

Depression does *not* lead to the motivation to care about self-care. An understanding health-care professional will be able to unload the diabetes care from the woman, allowing her to have more energy to cope with her other problems. Perhaps even a few sessions with a psychologist to learn coping skills would be helpful.

Exercise can be the perfect prescription for this depression. Exercise reverses the midline bulge, increases energy levels, and produces endorphins. Endorphins are naturally occurring brain substances that make us feel happy. These substances are responsible for the "runner's high," a feeling of euphoria much like the feeling one gets from taking an upper, or pep pill. In addition, exercise burns sugar and can therefore be used to improve glucose control.

JUNE AND BARBARA: Your exercise prescription is one we take daily and when we skip it, we feel much the worse for it. As card-carrying *troisième* agers, we'll tell what our usual routine is. (For once this is not a case of don't do as I do, do as I say, but rather it's "Do as I do.")

Our program is a three-pronged attack on decrepitude—and so far it's working. The three prongs are: stretching, strength training, and aerobics.

**Stretching.** This we do every day. We learned its importance the hard way—or at least Barbara did. During June's twenty-fifth diabetes anniversary Barbara always carried over her shoulder a bag heavy with vital necessities including all June's diabetes supplies, coffee-making equipment and coffee, manifold snacks, and cosmetics. Near the end of the year she started getting back pains, sometimes so intense she could hardly heave her legs out of bed in the morning. It was discovered she'd thrown herself out of whack with all that bag carrying. Several chiropractic treatments later, she was functioning pretty well in the back department, but not wanting to ever experience that pain and virtual immobility again. She started on a daily program of stretching exercises and has been doing them ever since. The back pain has never returned. Of course, she doesn't carry heavy bags over her shoulder now, always using a roll-on. Neither does she carry heavy purses on her shoulder, but instead she goes for the new stylish backpack. This is highly recommended for you, as it balances the weight and doesn't throw your back out of kilter. June, who knows how to profit from another's mistake, adopted the stretching exercises as preventive maintenance. For a complete guide to stretching we heartily recommend a book with the logical title: *Stretching*, by Bob Anderson (see Recommended Reading: Exercise). We each have selected our own favorite exercises from this, the ones that make us feel better—and we're sure you'll select yours.

Along with the stretching we do some leg lifts and sit-ups to strengthen the stomach muscles—very important for *troisième* agers who tend to expand in the stomach department (have you noticed?). Strengthening the stomach muscles also helps the back.

**Strength Training:** This is what you can do in a gym on those Nautilus and Cybex machines. You will, of course, need a lot of instruction and supervision in their use. If you don't feel you have an adequate supply of both of these commodities at your gym, change gyms. We worked out in a gym for a couple of years and liked it, but when our time got more and more and limited and the gym more and more crowded, we started doing hand weights at home. This means we don't get the leg workout we did on the machines at the gym, but we figure the upper-body strengthening is what we—and all women—need most, anyway. As a side benefit, upper-body strengthening, wherever you do it, promotes a youthful aura. Helen Gurley Brown, *Cosmopolitan*'s perennially almost preternaturally youthful editor, says that the best indicator of a woman's aging is loose flesh in the upper arm. Strength training with weights can make this indicator less indicative.

We started with three-pound weights, and after about a year June is up to five and Barbara (the queen of overdo) is up to eight. Following are the weight-training exercises we do. We do these every other day so the muscles will have a chance to repair themselves between sessions. (For an inexpensive and undemanding way to get started with strength training, see Dr. Lois's recommendations for exercises for pregnant women on pp. 242–245).

Note: Both the stretching and the weight training at home can get a tad boring, so when doing these, we keep our minds active by listening to *Morning Edition* on National Public Radio or studying languages on tapes.

**Aerobics:** Previously this meant jogging for us, but jogging is getting a bad press because of all the jarring of the knees, which is particularly not recommended for *troisième* agers. Now it's walking. Walking is an activity that most people enjoy, that doesn't take any special equipment—except well-fitting walking shoes—and that doesn't cause physical damage. Its benefits are tremendous.

Dr. Lawrence Power sang the praises of walking in his syndicated column: "A group of overweight volunteers were placed on restricted diets of 1,000 calories a day. Half were put on a 30-minute-a-day walking program; the other half were not . . . All subjects were measured at the start and finish for total body fat and muscle. The walking group had gained two pounds of muscle and lost 25 pounds of fat. The nonwalking group had lost eight pounds of muscle and 12 pounds of fat."

Dr. Power also pointed out that the diet-only group gained back weight much more easily, because of their smaller muscle mass, than the diet-and-exercise group. That's because muscle is a "metabolically busy" tissue and burns more calories than fat.

We walk as much as possible and whenever possible. You just can't walk too much, at least we never have. Every time we travel we try to stay on our feet almost all day, almost every day. Walking, to be aerobic, has to be more than a stroll or a saunter. The recommended pace is what is called "at conversational intensity." That is to say, you can talk while you walk without getting winded. (If you can sing while you walk, you're walking too slowly.) Gradually you'll be able to increase your conversational intensity speed until you reach the ultimate goal of the fifteen-minute mile—definitely a brisk pace. Our dream is to take a walking tour in Italy walking from town to town (with someone carting our luggage from hotel to hotel for us). We're calling this our "Walk for Pasta Tour." The more you walk, the more you can eat!

If you don't feel up to anything even as mildly strenuous as the activities described above, or if you have physical problems that preclude these activities, please don't give up on the idea of exercise. There are sitting-in-a-chair exercises that almost anyone can do, and there are videos available that show you how to do them (contact CC-M Productions, 8501 Cedar Street, Silver Spring, MD 20910; phone 800-453-6280). Any exercise you can do without pain or risk is far, far better than no exercise.

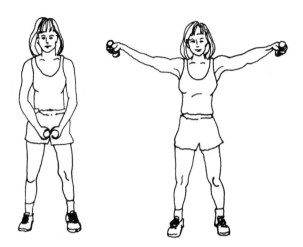

*Figure 4* **Side Shoulder Raise (outer portion of the shoulder).**
Start with your arms hanging in front of your thighs, elbows slightly
bent, and palms facing each other. Raise both dumbbells outward
simultaneously to shoulder height, keeping elbows slightly bent.
Lower dumbbells to starting position and repeat.

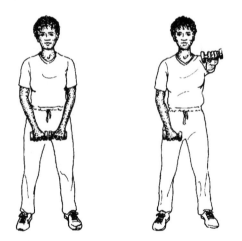

*Figure 5* **Front Shoulder Raise (front portion of the shoulder).** Begin with your arms hanging in front of your thighs and your
palms facing the thighs. Raise one dumbbell straight in front of you
to shoulder height. Lower this dumbbell to your starting position and
repeat using your other arm. Keep alternating your arms.

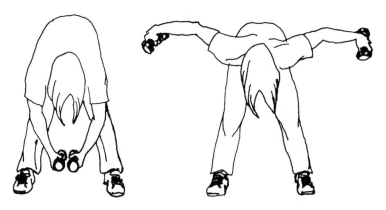

*Figure 6* **BENT-OVER SHOULDER RAISE (REAR PORTION OF THE SHOULDER AND UPPER BACK).** Bend over until your torso is roughly parallel to floor. Keep your knees slightly bent. Start with your arms hanging down toward the floor, palms facing inward, and elbows slightly bent. Raise both dumbbells outward simultaneously to shoulder height, keeping your elbows slightly bent. Lower the dumbbells to starting position and repeat.

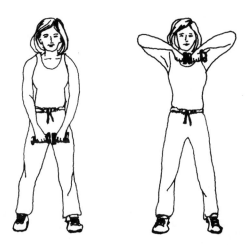

*Figure 7* **UPRIGHT ROW (SHOULDER, NECK, AND UPPER BACK).** Stand with your arms hanging in front of your thighs, palms facing your thighs, and the dumbbells close together. Keeping your palms close to the body, raise the dumbbells simultaneously to your chin. Lower the dumbbells to starting position and repeat.

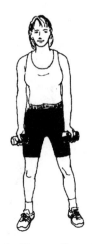
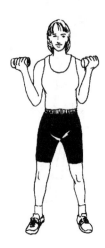

*Figure 8* **Biceps Curl (biceps, or front of upper arm).** Start the exercise with your arms hanging at your sides and your palms facing in front of you. Keeping the elbows close to the sides of the body, curl both dumbbells upward to the shoulders. Lower and repeat.

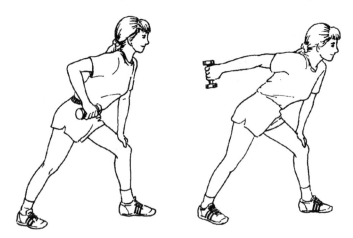

*Figure 9* **Triceps Extension (triceps, or back of upper arm).** Place one foot about a step in front of the other and bend both knees slightly. Lean forward and rest one hand, palm down, on the knee of your front leg. Place the hand with the dumbbell in it against your hip (palm of your hand facing the hip). Keeping your elbow still, straighten your arm fully. Then bend your arm until it returns to your hip and repeat. After completing the desired number of repetitions, repeat with the other arm.

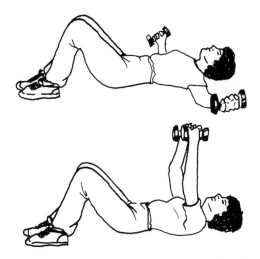

*Figure 10* **SUPINE FLY (CHEST MUSCLES).** Lie faceup on the floor. Place your arms perpendicular to your body. Raise both dumbbells up above your chest to meet in the center. Lower the dumbbells and repeat.

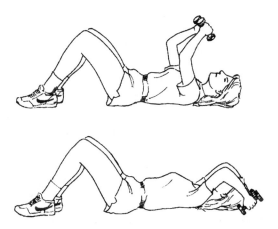

*Figure 11* **PULLOVER (CHEST AND BACK).** Lie faceup on the floor. Begin with the dumbbells held together directly above the center of your chest, with your elbows slightly bent. Lower the dumbbells to the floor behind your head, keeping your elbows bent. Raise the dumbbells back to starting position and repeat.

You'll find that exercise is like eating peanuts: it's hard to stop once you get started. You'll want to keep it up and keep feeling fit and euphoric for the rest of your life. You may even drift into what we call the whipped cream on top of the exercise sundae: sports. Pick something you really enjoy, like tennis or golf or swimming, and that will serve to augment and enhance your exercise program.

Dr. Lois, are there any special tips that you have for the exercising diabetic woman?

DR. LOIS: She should measure her blood sugar before the exercise program to ensure that it is in the 100 to 180 mg/dl range. Starting an exercise program with a blood sugar of much lower than 100 does not leave room to burn up sugar. Either the exercise should be rescheduled for the next day and the insulin dose decreased, or twenty grams of carbohydrate should be eaten.

On the other hand, exercising when the blood sugar is high only makes the sugar go higher. There may not be enough insulin on board to prevent the rise that may occur from the stress of exercise when the blood sugar is high. The concern is that a high blood sugar may become a dangerously higher blood sugar.

The above advice does not apply to those diabetic women who are able to manage their diabetes with pills or diet alone. In the case of these women with Type II diabetes, they may exercise no matter what their blood sugar levels are because they do not have trouble with swift plunges of glucose or life-threatening high blood sugars.

JUNE AND BARBARA: One woman wrote us asking for information on heart disease, saying, "Some troublesome symptoms I experienced for some time were mistakenly attributed by my doctor to bouts of low blood sugar. (When I began testing blood-sugar levels, I found this was *not* so!) Then, almost by serendipity, I found that the chest pains and irregular heart were due to a not-so-innocent mitral valve prolapse [MVP]. MVP is usually considered 'harmless,' whereas the version I have is a progressive form that greatly increases the work of the heart."

Is the mitral valve prolapse likely to have been caused by her diabetes?

DR. LOIS: Mitral valve prolapse is a separately inherited disease. Thus, the woman who wrote this letter inherited both MVP and diabetes mellitus. Diabetes does cause premature atherosclerosis, however, when the sugar level is sustained above normal for years. In fact, the usual statement is that diabetes "equalizes" the prevalence of atherosclerotic causes of heart attack. In other words, a diabetic woman would have the same chances of having a heart attack at the same age as a nondiabetic man. A nondiabetic woman has only a 5 percent chance of having a heart attack before menopause, whereas a woman who has had diabetes for more than thirty years has a 50 percent chance of this.

JUNE AND BARBARA: Those are rather discouraging statistics, but we've always had the theory that diabetes can, in some ways, be beneficial to your health. For example, a fifty-year-old diabetic woman who understands healthy living and takes good care of herself could conceivably be in better shape than a twenty-year-old nondiabetic who's let herself go to pot through ignorance and sloth. Have you seen evidence of this in your practice?

DR. LOIS: Unfortunately, I have seen unfit, fat women who can barely climb a flight of steps without becoming short of breath. But fortunately, I have seen many diabetic women over the age of fifty who are fit and the picture of health. I have personally met two elderly women who received the Joslin Medal for fifty years of diabetes with no evidence of any complications. Any of our readers who have had diabetes for fifty years and who are in good health should apply for the medal. (Write to the Joslin Diabetes Foundation, 50 Joslin Road, Boston, MA 02215.)

# 3 ❧ Both Sides Now

*Oh wad some power the giftie gie us*
*To see oursels as others see us!*

— R O B E R T   B U R N S

NOW THAT WE'VE LOOKED AT THE PICTURE OF DIABETES from your point of view, we're going to "gie you the giftie" of seeing it from the perspective of those close to a diabetic woman. We hope that their words will help you to help your family and friends come to terms with situations that may hurt and disturb them as much as— or more than—they hurt and disturb you. We suggest that after reading these sections, you pass them on to the appropriate people in your life.

Dr. Peterson (Dr. Jovanovic's husband), who tells the following story, is an eminent endocrinologist and coauthor of *The Diabetes Self-Care Method.*

# Love, Life, and the Pursuit of Happiness with a Diabetic Woman

*Charles M. Peterson, M.D.*

What happens when the woman you love has diabetes? Well, if it occurs during your relationship, you tend to deny it until that doesn't work, then you get angry and ask, "Why us?" and finally you begin to acquire better coping skills—but only after a time of real depression.

How can two people who have been to medical school and who specialize in diabetes deny that one of them has the disease? Easily. It hurts too much to accept it all at once, no matter how "smart" you may be. The hurt does not go away very soon, either.

One of the best things that families in which someone has developed diabetes can do is talk with someone about the experience and about diabetes itself. The format is almost not as important as the process, since talking helps overcome denial and helps move the family through the stages of grief into the real world of coping. Unfortunately, the male of the species is less apt to talk with others about the real hurts of life and more likely to keep them inside. In addition, his soul mate is the one with diabetes—and he feels it would be better if it were he. Certainly, it is easier to cope with your own infirmities—physical and spiritual— than with those of the one you love.

Which brings us to the next problem: a man likes action; he likes to fix things and make them right—preferably *now*. Yet there is no way for a man to fix his partner's diabetes. He has to let her grow, make mistakes, and suffer with her own diabetes without interfering with the process and yet be there to discuss, support, and learn with her. It is difficult to let go of children so they can grow, but it is even more difficult to let go of a spouse who has a chronic illness. Diabetes is a time of taking hold and setting free, just like marriage itself.

Yet you *can* take away some of your own anxiety so that you can help your partner in more and deeper ways. Anxiety comes from the unknown, so learn to cope with diabetes. (It will take a lifetime to learn to cope with your partner anyway, so start with the diabetes—it's easier!) Learn about measuring blood sugar. Practice on yourself. Learn about injections by giving yourself injections of sterile saline [salt solution]. Learn how to inject glucagon to bring her out of a hypoglycemic episode, and have a plan to ensure that you will always have glucagon available where both of you can find it. Once in Italy I did the world's fastest and messiest unpacking job at 3 A.M., because we were too lazy to locate the glucagon before going to bed after the flight from the United States. It took us about two hours to get the room in shape the next morning so we wouldn't be embarrassed when the maid saw it.

Learn about food and the carbohydrate count of various foods so that you can help her count carbos, and you will both begin to have a healthier eating pattern. Learn about exercise (strength training, cardiovascular conditioning, and flexibility) and start a program for both of you.

Families get stronger from coping with challenges. Cope with the challenge of diabetes as a family. If you seem to be stuck, get a consultation from a professional. Above all, keep learning, growing, and challenging each other so that you as a family are taking charge of diabetes and winning over it—with love.

**JUNE AND BARBARA:** We've seen the truth of all of Dr. Peterson's words in action. Amy's husband, Michael, became such an expert in diabetes during her pregnancy that now whenever he meets someone in his business who has diabetes in the family, he gives them an instant education. He takes a great deal of pride in being able to help others in this way. And we've often seen how the health and vitality of a family improve when the whole family adopts the lifestyle of its diabetic member.

Unfortunately, not all husbands are like Dr. Peterson and Michael, as this letter from Karen Kremsreiter in Baraboo, Wisconsin, points out.

My husband was very supportive. He read every piece of literature I brought home and helped me figure out dietary calculations. He learned how to give me shots in places I thought I couldn't reach. (I've since learned to inject myself anywhere.) He learned how to use glucagon and often recognized signs of an insulin reaction long before I did. Looking back (I'm forty years old now), I feel that my husband's support and involvement were critical in my ability to become confident and adept in diabetes management.

Although he is no longer so intensely involved with my routine, he is still willing to listen and learn. That means that there is one person (aside from my doctor) with whom I can have an intelligent conversation about diabetes and who understands the fine points of diabetes management.

The reason I mention my husband's support is that I see this kind of support lacking among the majority of diabetic women I meet. When a diabetes support group started in my town about ten years ago, I was eager to join. My husband went to meetings with me, and we both learned a lot. However, we were surprised to find so few men at these meetings. I assumed that there weren't many diabetic men in my town (wrong!) or that some of the elderly women were widowed (wrong again!).

Eventually, I became chairman of the diabetes group, which gave me the chance to get to know the members well. Over the years, the patterns have remained pretty much the same. Husbands generally do not attend meetings with their diabetic wives. However, wives usually do attend with their diabetic husbands, or wives attend FOR their husbands or diabetic children. The woman, it seems, is still considered the primary caretaker of the health of all family members.

The sad part of this pattern is that women who have supportive husbands (or sisters or friends) do much better, healthwise. The diabetic women who attend meetings alone seem to have many more complaints about stress. They worry that their diabetes is "inconveniencing" their husbands and families. They require more trips to the doctor and need to ask for rides to meetings they wish to attend. Many of these women seem to develop complications of diabetes sooner.

Women need to be convinced that they never have to apologize to anyone for having diabetes. Moreover, they should insist that another family member learn some fine points of diabetes care. Type II diabetes, especially, is often glossed over as a mild, harmless disorder by other family members. It's time people realized that Type II diabetes can be as fatal as Type I diabetes when the home treatment is sloppy and inadequate. Diabetes care requires a lot of education and some special techniques, which all family members should be involved in. And a woman should not feel guilty for placing her health above other family problems.

Any suggestions you can make for involving husbands and family members in the diabetes management program would be helpful. Perhaps it is the family doctor who needs to be more aggressive in involving the entire family.

DR. LOIS: Mrs. Kremsreiter is correct about the fact that women who have support at home do better. Studies have clearly shown that when a husband and wife are in conflict about the diabetes, her hemoglobin $A_{1C}$ is the highest.

I also agree with her about the family doctor's responsibility for involving the family. He or she could use glucagon-injection education as a gimmick to force the husband to come into the office, and once he is there a bit of family therapy could be started. This should be followed up with an appointment with a real family therapist who is trained in diabetes.

JUNE AND BARBARA: Perhaps you could also provide us with a few guidelines on setting up a support group, so that women out there alone could actually initiate a network if none existed in the community.

DR. LOIS: That's very possible. Anyone can start a support group. When people with the same problems meet together spontaneously, things get better. Even without a professional counselor to guide discussions, the group process is helpful, because just living with diabetes means that coping skills have been developed. Thus an experienced person with diabetes can do wonders for a new diabetic.

The group can benefit, too, from a professionally trained person with skills in coping, but not having such an expert should in no way deter you from starting a support group.

JUNE AND BARBARA: Both you and Dr. Peterson point out the necessity of getting psychological help from a professional if you seem to be stuck. This is tremendously valid. We should all get rid of that old Sam Goldwyn idea that anybody who goes to a psychiatrist ought to have his head examined. No one should ever hesitate to seek psychological counseling when it's called for. Nancy Slonim Aronie, the mother of a diabetic child, gave a vivid example of how effective such counseling can be by relating the following personal experience on National Public Radio's program *All Things Considered.*

# The Night Mom Lost It at Friendly's

*Nancy Slonim Aronie*

I used to think I would never go to a psychologist. Psychologists were for the rich, the spoiled, and the bored, and, of course, the crazy. I prided myself on being none of these. Then when my nine-month-old son was diagnosed as diabetic, my life changed. His diabetes didn't make me rich, spoiled, or bored, but it almost made me crazy. I had to give him two shots of insulin a day in his tiny little arms. I had to collect his urine in little plastic bags and test it for sugar three times a day. I worried when he was napping that he would never wake up, and I worried in the middle of the night whether he had eaten enough before he went to sleep.

When he got a little older, other parents worried. He soon learned he held this terrible power. Grown-ups were afraid of him. They would ask him what he wanted, and if he needed to rest, and if he were thirsty, and what should they make special for him when he was coming over to play with their children. He didn't like this power, and they didn't like having a kid visiting who might die on them any minute. His invitations were limited. As parents we tried very hard not to indulge him . . . to treat him like a "normal" person. But every so often we blew it.

One night after a concert we took our two kids out to Friendly's and he asked for ice cream. I said no. My husband said, "Oh, let him have ice cream."

"LET HIM?!" I screamed, "Oh, I get it. *I'm* in charge of the pancreas. *I* can make it work. *I'm* the bad guy here, and you're the good guy. Poor Dan. He never gets a treat, and it's my fault."

At this point in my life I had many psychologist friends who had erased the myth that therapy was lying on a couch once a week for fourteen years while a Freudian-looking shrink with pencil poised in hand nodded and told you all your problems stemmed from the fact that you were really in love with your father, hated your mother, and wished you were your brother. So I called a few of my friends and said, "This diabetes thing has gotten out of hand. Dan is angry all the time, and I am guilty all the time, and we need help. Whom should we go see?"

I got a name, and within a week the four of us were sitting in an office in four big leather chairs in a circle.

The doctor asked my eleven-year-old son, "Why are you here?"

"I think it's because of the night my mom lost it at Friendly's," he said.

The doctor turned to my nine-year-old, the one with diabetes, and said, "Why do *you* think you're here?"

My nine-year-old smiled and said, "Yup, that's it. It was the night my mom lost it at Friendly's."

And then he turned to my husband, who had fought tooth and nail not to go to this appointment. My husband nodded in agreement. "Yeah. We're here because Nance made us come."

Then the doctor turned to me. I reached for the box of Kleenex on his desk and burst into tears. I said, "We're here because this child thinks the world is going to change its rules for him because he has diabetes. *He* gets four strikes in baseball, not three. And this child, who doesn't have diabetes, is wounded because all of the focus has been on the other one. And this man, my husband, doesn't want a child with diabetes because it hurts too much. So I'm the only one who has a son with diabetes, and they all think I control the pancreas, and, please, could you shape us up in short order?"

The doctor smiled and asked some key questions. We told a story of how one night before a fancy party I had prepared my son with a lecture on how there would be all these tempting foods, telling him that he should have a small amount of everything so that he wouldn't feel deprived.

The first person to grab a plate was my son, and when I saw the huge mound of sweet-potato pudding he had taken, I said, "Dan, I thought we had talked about having small portions of everything."

"This IS small!" he screamed, then smashed the plate down and ran out of the room crying.

The doctor gave a great analogy. He said to Dan, "If you were describing a quarter to a kid who was poor and you were describing the same quarter to a kid who was rich, how would the rich kid's understanding of the size of the quarter be different from the poor kid's?"

Dan said, "Well, the rich kid would see the quarter smaller because a quarter isn't much money to him, but to a poor kid a quarter is a lot so it would be bigger."

"Exactly," said the doctor. "Well, to your mom, who worries about your health because she loves you, the amount of sweet-potato pudding was a lot, but to you, who never has enough, the pudding portion was small."

I saw my son understand. I saw the switch go on. I saw him see that all I was doing was loving him and worrying about him, not trying to make his life miserable.

The next session we talked about his anger. The doctor

said, "Your mom didn't give you diabetes. She's sorry you have diabetes. It's not fair, but life isn't fair. Your mom is not in charge of your pancreas. Neither is your father or your brother. Being angry is okay, but choose where the anger goes. Your mother is hurting, and she loves you. Being angry at her is not going to make the diabetes go away."

Another click. Another light. A few more sessions and the doctor told us to go home and to call if we had a crisis or just wanted to come in and talk.

Now there is harmony in my house except for the usual teenage growing-up stuff, and I realize what a luxury it is to be able to go and talk to a pro and get perspective so simply, so easily, so quickly. It takes work. It takes commitment (and a willingness to change and to hear some truths), but you don't have to be rich, spoiled, bored, or crazy—and you can even go talk to someone *before* you lose it at Friendly's.

This story shows the problems a mother can have in coping with her child's diabetes, but probably the most difficult moment for the mother comes when the child—particularly a very young child—is diagnosed as diabetic. What do you say and do to help a mother at this time?

DR. LOIS: I have thought about this question for a long while, because my experience with mothers of diabetic children is limited. As you know, I am an internist, which means that I take care of adults. My youngest patients are twelve years old, but I treat them as adults, and my interaction with their parents is minimal.

Yes, I have given numerous lectures to parents of diabetic children, but this formal setting does not lend itself to answering intimate questions. Usually these parent groups are composed of experienced parents who just want to learn more about diabetes research. I really could not answer this question with the voice of experience until just recently, when I came face-to-face with it on a very personal level.

A childhood friend of mine with whom I had not communicated for years called me up. She is a very special person of whom I was always envious. She succeeded in becoming the prima ballerina of the New York City Ballet Company, whereas I was too short and too awkward to make it as a ballerina, so I became a doctor. Not only is she truly talented and exquisitely beautiful, but she is also blessed with a beautiful personality. This is all to tell you that there never was a more perfect woman created. Why, then, did diabetes strike her one-year-old daughter?

Two weeks before she telephoned me, her daughter had been taken to the hospital in diabetic coma. I heard her pain and grief. Her emotions were mixed with anger and disbelief. To make matters worse, no one at the hospital helped her to cope, grieve, and begin to accept. No one told her what diabetes is, what it meant for her daughter, and what the best management program is. My friend left the hospital with her daughter out of coma, but with no understanding of how to give insulin and how to prepare meals. I just listened and grieved with her. It is quite possible that the best diabetes educator tediously went over all the basics, but one thing is sure. The week the little one is on the critical list is no time to try to teach skills that take complete attention.

My response was not to take sides but instead to offer a sympathetic ear. No, God was not punishing her. Goodness knows that she, of all people, did not deserve punishment. Yet her sense of guilt was real, and my job was to tell her over and over that diabetes occurs spontaneously. If sin caused diabetes, it would be easier to cure.

My next job was to direct her to support systems. I referred her to a specialized center for children with diabetes that has a team whose members are expert on the problems children face. The dietitian is skilled in baby food, the psychologist knows how to handle baby problems, and the diabetes doctor knows baby metabolism. In addition, my friend could meet other mothers and share experiences. She could also take classes to learn more about diabetes. This would help her not to feel so inadequate.

My last job was to reassure her that I was overjoyed about renewing our friendship and that I was here for her. Too often, friends tend to shy away when there are problems, and it is at this time that support is most needed.

A week later my friend called me again. Her voice was full of hope. She had learned insulin action, and her fear of hypoglycemia was not constantly present. She had learned how to do blood tests to prevent hypoglycemia, and she had learned how to treat hypoglycemia. She then confessed that her fear of hypoglycemia was greater than her fear of the diagnosis of diabetes. The psychologist solved this problem easily. The dietitian spoke in ways that made sense for feeding a year-old baby. The diabetes doctor developed better doses of insulin, which matched the eating and sleeping patterns of a small child. Life seemed better. But I explained to my friend that accepting the diagnosis of diabetes takes at least a year and that it certainly is not an indulgence to grieve.

JUNE AND BARBARA: You mentioned the anger of your friend over her child's diabetes. We see this all the time. In fact, we find that possibly the angriest people on the face of the earth are the mothers of diabetic children. In his book *Feeling Good*, Dr. David Burns writes that one of the greatest sources of anger is the feeling that a situation is unfair. And what could be more unfair than having your innocent child, who has never done anything to anyone, be diagnosed as diabetic? Psychoanalyst Willard Gaylen believes that one cause of anger is the feeling of not having control over a situation. Both are probably right.

A big problem with anger, however, is that diabetics and parents of diabetics often don't like to admit, even to themselves, that the source of their anger is diabetes. So they displace their anger, directing it toward something or someone else. You may have experienced this yourself. Perhaps you have suddenly become furious over the time you've had to spend in the waiting room, over the doctor's bill, about the meter that reads a high number, or even with the well-meaning and compassionate health professional who is trying to help you make changes that you don't want to make. This last is a prime cause of burnout and compassion fatigue among diabetes health professionals. Even though they try to understand the reasons behind your anger, it really breaks their hearts and spirits when you suddenly and without provocation bite their helping hands.

The worst thing about displacing your anger—even worse than the psychic damage you do to a hapless "displacee"—is that if you never admit the true source of your anger, you'll never get rid of it. It will keep festering and then erupting. As Gaylen puts it, "Expressing anger is a form of public littering . . . how futile and how dangerous it is." He also shoots down the idea that it's therapeutic to let off steam by blowing up. It is far better to permanently resolve the situation that is the source of your anger. Again, some kind of therapy may be needed to do this.

The one good thing we can say about anger is that it's

a step up from depression, which some experts regard as inner-directed anger and an even harder problem to deal with.

Another prime source of anger and also of resentment (which we have heard defined as a demand that someone feel guilty) is the situation in which one member of the family, such as a child, has diabetes, and the others do not. Should everyone be made to eat only what the diabetic child can? Should the child's brothers and sisters just ignore the diabetes? How much special attention should the diabetic child get?

DR. LOIS: The brothers and sisters of a diabetic child should not be deprived of the delights of cakes, candies, sodas, chocolates, and ice cream. All too often, if siblings are denied things, they become angry and resentful of the diabetic child. Perhaps it is better to teach the diabetic child about the real world, which is full of forbidden foods, but to do so gently. For example, I usually suggest that whenever the family is on an outing and the other kids get an ice cream cone, the child with diabetes could have an alternative snack (yogurt, hot dog, popcorn) and should also get an extra treat—say, a toy—that the others do *not* get.

All of the brothers and sisters should be taught to be comfortable with diabetes, needles, and blood tests. The diabetes should not be hidden from the rest of the family; rather, the process of diabetes care should be shared. I like to suggest that the premeal blood-glucose strip be read visually by all the other children, with the one who reads it closest to the meter reading getting something special.

Many times the other brothers and sisters feel left out and are in fact jealous of the doted-on diabetic child. Here, the mother needs to be sensitive to these feelings, and she should try to spend as much special time with each of the other children as she does with the diabetic child.

The hardest job for Mom is not to be overly protective. Except for insulin injections, a diabetic child is no different physically or mentally from other children, and he or she should therefore not be treated as a crippled person. Too often the child will succumb to a lazy dependence, and the growing-up process becomes more difficult than it ought to be. The mother needs to be brave, allowing the child independence and the right to make mistakes. Gentle guidance can be used to right the wrong and reinforce the right. I guess we are asking Mom to be a saint—but after all, diabetes only happens to the best people!

JUNE AND BARBARA: It's important for parents of diabetic children to go out in order to get out from under the strain of caring for a diabetic child. However, they often worry all evening that the baby-sitter won't know what to do if there's a crisis. Do you have any suggestions for them?

DR. LOIS: I've heard of parents of diabetic children doing baby-sitting trade-offs with parents of other diabetic children. I think this is a super idea. Then they can go out with confidence, knowing that their child is in the hands of someone who understands diabetes as only the parent of a diabetic child can. Diabetic moms make great baby-sitters, too!

JUNE AND BARBARA: Some mothers who have diabetes wonder what they should tell their children about diabetes. Could you share with us your personal experience with your own children?

**DR. LOIS:** My children need to accept me for what I am—a woman with diabetes. My diabetes doesn't make me unfair, dishonest, selfish, or uncaring. Yes, it does mean that I am less than perfect, and my children either love me anyway or they don't. The simplest thing to tell you is that if I am embarrassed about my diabetes, then so are my children. If I am open about my diabetes and make it a natural part of life, then I should not be surprised that my kids tell strangers that their mommy has diabetes. Not only are they not embarrassed, but they may also even be proud because Mom is somehow special, or they may feel that they are special because they have so much medical background at a young age.

Fourteen years ago I was invited to give a talk to first-year medical students to help in trying to create a new generation of doctors who would be more open to diabetes self-care. These med students were fresh out of college and probably didn't even know what insulin was. My five- and six-year-old children were not yet in school and my baby-sitter was sick, so I took my children to the lecture and sat them in the back with strict orders to be quiet.

I started the lecture and fell into my usual jargon of medicalese. I noted that the class was unruly, but I kept right up with my rushed pace in order to pack in as much information as possible, using the longest words. I spotted my six-year-old son walking down the aisle and climbing onto the stage. I continued to talk, but boy, was I mad! My son marched up to the podium and said, "Mommy, no one understands you. The people around me are muttering that they don't know what diabetes is." I turned to my son and began my lecture over again. This time I tried to explain myself so *he* would understand. Every time I accidentally used a big word, he would stop me and ask for an explanation. At the end of the talk, he received a standing ovation. Then he joined me every year and we reenacted this routine, to the joy of the students.

How did he know so much? How did he know where I should put the emphasis and what is important to teach? He knew because he grew up with a mom who has diabetes and who is open to him about needles and blood tests and about what to expect when I am hypo-glycemic. When I have low blood sugar, I get irritated for no reason. He now knows me well enough not to ask, "Are you low?" because he knows that I will say, "I am NOT LOW." Instead, he asks me to do simple arithmetic. I happen to be quick at mental gymnastics, and if I have trouble with 99 minus 13, then even I will admit that I must be low. If I need him to help me eat or get food, he knows exactly what to do.

Teaching the children about diabetes is an everyday process and makes mothering special.

JUNE AND BARBARA: Novelist and philosopher Aldous Huxley spent his entire life in pursuit of knowledge. In his later years someone asked him, considering all his scholarship and deep thought, what philosophical con-clusion he had reached. He paused. "I think," he said slowly, "it's just that we should all be a little kinder to one another."

The caring kindness given to a diabetic woman by those closest to her enriches their lives as much as it enriches hers. But perhaps those closest aren't certain what kind of special kindnesses a woman needs. We have the answer to that. Our favorite expert on how to live with a diabetic is Dr. Richard Rubin. He is our collabo-rator on the book *Psyching Out Diabetes*. Dr. Rubin has a diabetic sister and son and has been counseling in the field of diabetes for over twenty years at Johns Hopkins Medical School and Hospital and in his private practice. Here are his words of wisdom:

## Ten Commandments for Avoiding Negative Scenes with Diabetic Loved Ones:

### 1. Thou Shalt Not Act like a Policeperson.

This approach doesn't work and can ruin your relationship.

### 2. Thou Shalt Not Ignore Diabetes.

Don't expect your loved one to carry on all activities as if the diabetes did not exist.

### 3. Thou Shalt Not Lead Your Loved One in the Paths of Temptation.

Many diabetics find it upsetting to be constantly face-to-face with forbidden fruits, and they often get angry at the person who's eating those fruits in front of them.

### 4. Thou Shalt Not Criticize When Your Loved One Succumbs to Temptation.

Sure, you're frustrated, but adding insult to injury is a surefire argument starter.

### 5. Thou Shalt Not Talk about Your Loved One's Diabetes in Public Unless Invited to Do So.

Public comments tend to be taken as criticism, so take your cue from your loved one.

## 6. Thou Shalt Offer Support and Comfort, Especially When Things Aren't Going Well with the Diabetes.

For any number of reasons, diabetics are often very touchy when their control is bad. A little extra TLC goes a long way toward avoiding confrontations at these times.

## 7. Thou Shalt Have the Patience of a Saint When Your Loved One Is Acutely Hypo- or Hyperglycemic.

These can be the worst of times, and if you both lose your heads . . . More on this issue later.

## 8. Thou Shalt Deal Constructively with Your Own Natural Fears and Resentments.

Your diabetic loved one is not the only one living with the disease. You are, too, and you will feel scared, angry, even overwhelmed at times. You must find a way to deal with these feelings constructively, on your own and with your loved one. The key is to acknowledge what you're feeling and to take responsibility for the feeling.

## 9. Thou Shalt Be Especially Sensitive in Public Situations.

Eating right, testing, and taking shots can be especially stressful for diabetics in public settings, so your diabetic loved one might be edgier than usual. Be alert for opportunities to make things a little easier.

## 10. Thou Shalt Find Out What Works and Do It.

In your family, a number of diabetes-related situations may often lead to conflict; for instance, when your loved one has high blood sugar, eats something he or she shouldn't, or fights you when you want to help him or her deal with an insulin reaction. Find out what your loved one wants you to do in these situations, and do it. Don't wait until you're in the middle of a battle to ask, though. Ask when you're both feeling comfortable and relaxed. I never cease to be amazed at how well this simple approach works to avoid fights.

# 4 ⚜ *D*iabetic Diet
## à la Carte

IN USING THIS TITLE, WE'RE NOT JUST CONTINUING WITH the French motif. We're also pointing out a major change in the diabetic's eating plan. Back in the bad old days, every diabetic was handed a one-sheet exchange list of permitted foods—the diabetic menu. No substitutions. No variations. No accounting for individual tastes or ethnic preferences. The list was both boring and limited, and it was little wonder that most diabetics decided to forget the whole thing and just go back to eating what they wanted.

Mercifully, the boring, rigid menu for diabetics is gone forever. In fact, there was a dramatic breakthrough in 1994 when the American Diabetes Association announced new dietary guidelines so simplifying and liberalizing diabetic eating that the present seems pure joy compared with the restrictions of the past. Instead of the same set ratios of protein, fat, and carbohydrate for everyone, each person is to have an individualized meal plan tailored to her diabetes type, body weight, exercise patterns, life circumstance, and personal tastes. The rec-ommendation is simply that protein should make up 10 to 20 percent of your calories and the remaining 80 to 90 percent be divided between fats and carbohydrates, de-pending on your own weight concerns and particular health risks such as cholesterol and triglycerides. The amount of carbohydrate you eat is considered more im-portant than the kind.

And that brings us to the most spectacular change. Sugar is now allowed in small amounts and is counted as a carbohydrate exchange. For example, one carbohy-drate exchange could be half a banana or half a cup of mashed potatoes or 1 tablespoon of sugar. From this you see that you still don't eat a whole bunch of sugar or you wouldn't have enough other food to fill you up and give you good nutrition. It's better to enjoy your smattering of sugar in something like ice cream because its fat con-tent slows down the entrance of sugar into the blood-stream. It is for this reason that Dr. Lois allows ice cream as a bedtime snack for pregnant diabetic women.

All this means that it finally is truly possible to dine à la carte, choosing what pleases you, adjusting the dia-betic diet to yourself rather than adjusting yourself to the diabetic diet. You do have to know what you're do-ing, though. An investment in learning that will really pay off is to have a session or two with a registered dieti-tian—preferably one who is a Certified Diabetes Educa-tor—who can help you create an eating plan that is compatible with both your taste and the requirements of your diabetes and your general health. To find a dieti-tian, try contacting the local chapter of your ADA, a local hospital with a diabetes program, or call the Ameri-can Dietetic Association's division of Dietitians in Dia-betes Care and Education, 1-800-877-1600, extension

4815 or the American Association of Diabetes Educators, 1-800-DMED.

Armed with this knowledge, you can play infinite variations on your own personal diabetic meal-plan theme. Appendix A lists an array of cookbooks that show you how to dine like a gourmet, feast like a queen, and enjoy all manner of international cuisines.

In case you don't have access to a dietitian to get you started down the right gastronomic paths, we'll ask Dr. Lois to first give you advice on that major dietary problem, weight loss or weight gain, as well as a brief rundown on the basics of the best kinds of eating plans for the different types of diabetes. Then we'll follow up with some tips of our own.

JUNE AND BARBARA: Women in our society are, unfortunately, overly concerned with their weight for appearance' sake. Along with the natural human tendency to want to look good in society's terms, diabetic women also have the need to keep their weight at a healthy level. Often, we see Type I women who need to put on a few pounds and Type II women who need to take off a few —or many—pounds. Why is there this difference? Let's take the Type I's first.

DR. LOIS: A Type I diabetic running high blood sugars usually has an intense feeling of hunger, known medically as polyphasia. The added calories she tends to eat at this time are usually lost into the urine. Therefore, classically out-of-control diabetes in an insulin-dependent woman is usually associated with cachexia (being markedly underweight).

Once the diabetes is brought under control, the calories no longer spill over into the urine. Instead, the body, with the help of insulin, stores the extra calories in the form of fat. Unfortunately, after a time of overeating, the natural habit will be to continue to overeat even if calories are no longer being lost into the urine. For that reason, you have to make a major effort to decrease caloric intake along with following any program of tightening blood-sugar control.

In addition, many women swell up when they come into better control. Diabetes out of control is associated with thirst from massive urination. Even though the massive urination stops when the diabetes is in better control, the habit to overdrink remains. Thus, an effort to decrease fluid intake to one quart a day helps prevent this swelling.

JUNE AND BARBARA: That's an important point about fluid intake. One Type I diabetic woman who got herself in good control was disturbed by abdominal bloating. What confused her—and us—was that she was not at all overweight, yet she had developed a distended stomach. Apparently, she had cut back on her calories to keep her weight normal, but she didn't realize that she was still drinking as many fluids as ever.

We hate to mention the following because we don't want to give anyone any bad ideas, but if a Type I diabetic woman wanted to lose weight she could just get out of control again by decreasing her insulin, and no matter what she ate she wouldn't gain weight.

DR. LOIS: Yes, the extra calories would automatically come out into the urine. This is what we call "diabetic anorexia," and it would be as damaging to the diabetic woman as the other anorexia—in fact, even more so. Not only would she have the poor health risks of being too thin, this terrible blood-sugar control would put her at risk for the horrifying complications of diabetes and, if carried to an extreme, for ketoacidosis and death.

When a woman is in good control, she realizes that it takes willpower to diet and exercise in order to stay fit. She also realizes that it's worth the effort, since her reward will be to look and feel wonderful now and to avoid complications later on in life.

JUNE AND BARBARA: How about the Type II women and their ongoing struggle to get weight off? The new nutritional guidelines do not pressure overweight Type II's to try for normal body weight that may be impossible to achieve and even more impossible to maintain. Their goal should be a "reasonable" weight. Losing only ten to twenty pounds may be enough to improve their diabetes control, and diabetes control, not weight loss should be their number-1 priority, according to the guidelines. Is there a way to help Type II women lose this weight so that they'll be in better control?

DR. LOIS: The treatment of choice is naturally to decrease food ingestion. Two hundred to 500 calories fewer than average would be a moderate daily restriction. But even this is not an easy treatment to carry out. Most Type II diabetic women became obese from an eating disorder to begin with. Since an eating disorder is involved, merely prescribing a reduction in calories is useless. A physician must provide: first, good educational support; second, a dietitian to translate the physician's prescription into meal planning; and third, psychological support—not only with trained psychologists specializing in eating disorders but also with group support such as Weight Watchers, Overeaters Anonymous, and so on, in which the patients help one another to sustain willpower. Physicians are not true to their patients if they think that all they need to do is write out a diet prescription and say, "See me in a month."

Every woman with an eating disorder needs help, whether or not she has diabetes and, if so, whether the diabetes is Type I or Type II. The best help is obtained by seeing a clinical psychologist trained in eating disorders and by attending group help sessions with peer input.

JUNE AND BARBARA: Weight loss is such a problem for many diabetic women that it would help a great deal if you could give a specific weight-loss program for Type I's and Type II's. We assume these programs would be different. Let's start with the Type I's.

DR. LOIS: For a Type I diabetic woman, the best way to go on a diet is to first become stabilized with the right amount of insulin to match the right amount of food for maintaining a steady body weight. Then, if the food intake is reduced by 25 percent, the insulin taken to cover the food can also be reduced by 25 percent. Let's say that the breakfast meal took eight units of Regular, lunch took four units of Regular, and dinner took eight units of Regular. If each meal were reduced by 25 percent, then breakfast would require six units of Regular, lunch three units of Regular, and dinner six units of Regular.

As far as diets are concerned, you have to be careful to *never* follow one of the popularized fad diets. These unbalanced "miracle weight-loss plans" that push one food—such as grapefruit—or one type of food (high protein, high fiber) to the exclusion of all others are bad enough for nondiabetics, but for diabetic people they are a disaster. The truth is that the only diets that produce a true weight reduction are those that cause you to lose the weight gradually by cutting the caloric intake below the caloric expenditure. (See Appendix A for recommended weight-loss books.)

To judge the amount of insulin needed, you must examine the particular diet, especially the amount of carbohydrate it contains. One unit of Regular insulin covers about 10 grams of carbohydrate. If food consists mostly of protein and fat, less insulin is needed. Fat does not need extra insulin to be metabolized. Protein is about 50 percent converted to glucose in about two or three hours. Therefore, protein usually is covered by the undercurrent basal insulin or the NPH or ultralente. Carbohydrate is covered by the mealtime Regular.

I'll try to give a formula for figuring this: say, for example, that a woman weighing 60 kilograms (approximately 132 pounds) needs 0.6 units per kilogram to maintain normal blood sugar, with half of this insulin needed as the basal requirement and half needed for meals. Then, if the twenty-four-hour insulin requirement is represented by $I$: $I$ = Basal + Mealtime Regular (or Basal = $\frac{1}{2}$ of $I$ and Meals = $\frac{1}{2}$ of $I$).

If the meals equal 1,800 calories (30 kcal × 60 kg) and 40 percent of this is carbohydrate, and if each gram of carbohydrate is 4 calories, then:

$$\frac{\text{Grams of Carbohydrate}}{24 \text{ Hours}} = \frac{1800 \times 40\%}{4 \text{ CAL/GM Carbohydrate}} \text{ or}$$
$$= 180 \text{ GM Carbohydrate per } 24\text{-Hour Period}$$

If the Mealtime Regular is Half of $I$, then:

$$\frac{60 \text{ KG} \times 0.6}{2} = 18 \text{ Units of Regular Cover } 180 \text{ Grams of Carbohydrate}$$

If the meals are divided equally, then each meal has sixty carbohydrates and requires six units of insulin. Now you see why one unit of regular covers ten grams of carbohydrate.

On a diet *before* weight loss, the basal is still half of *I* per eighteen units until weight is lost, but the meal Regular is decreased to intake. So if a person wants only twenty grams of carbohydrate for breakfast, she takes two units; for lunch, if she wants thirty grams of carbohydrate, she takes three units, and so on. Of course, a woman may find that for her one unit does not cover a full ten grams of carbohydrate, so she may need one unit for eight grams of carbohydrate. On the other hand, if she is sensitive to Regular, she may take one unit of Regular to cover twelve to fifteen grams of carbohydrate. With this match, food can be increased or decreased without hyperglycemia or hypoglycemia.

JUNE AND BARBARA: Is it as complicated for a Type II diabetic?

DR. LOIS: It's not as complicated, but it may be more difficult, because an overweight Type II may have "hungry fat cells" pleading for food all the time. The best plan is for these persons to have a constant support system. A program like Weight Watchers is most successful in giving support. Busy physicians are the worst support system, but they *are* needed to reduce the oral agents as needed while food intake and weight are decreased.

JUNE AND BARBARA: We've heard a lot lately about fat cells being responsible for overweight, and the current medical tendency is to blame mothers for overfeeding babies and causing more fat cells to develop. Has this been proven, or is it just another case of the mother getting a bum rap?

**DR. LOIS:** It hasn't yet been proven in humans, but they have discovered in laboratories that overfed baby rats develop more fat cells than their normally fed counterparts. Based on those studies, some researchers feel it would apply to people as well.

Other studies have found that overweight babies have larger-than-normal fat cells and also that very overweight adults have more than the normal number of fat cells. However, no one has yet discovered when this increase in fat cells occurs. They do know, however, that once a fat cell is formed, it's with you for life. It shrinks when you lose weight, but it's still there, fairly screaming with hunger. This helps to explain why people put back on as much weight as they have just lost or more. Their shrunken fat cells keep demanding food.

**JUNE AND BARBARA:** We have a friend, a home-economics professor, who maintains that she'd be a perfect candidate for survival of enforced starvation because her body stores fat so efficiently and burns it off so inefficiently. Is this a common problem among overweight people?

**DR. LOIS:** Yes, everyone's body has protective mechanisms that help protect it from starvation by changing the metabolism so that as much energy as possible is conserved. As soon as you cut back on food, the body adjusts itself to burning less.

**JUNE AND BARBARA:** What's the answer, then, for overweight Type II women who have large fat cells and/or a "starvation-survival" metabolism?

DR. LOIS: I'm afraid the answer is a dull one, and one you've heard a hundred times: a reduction in calories and an increase in exercise. Those weird crash diets may be easier to stick to because you figure you can stand anything for a brief period, but, almost invariably, as soon as the diet is over and the weight is lost you return to your old eating habits and put all the weight back on, usually with a few pounds' dividend. Not only that, but crash diets are usually unbalanced and unhealthy and therefore especially risky for a diabetic woman.

JUNE AND BARBARA: A lot of women hesitate to quit smoking because it's almost axiomatic that you put on weight when you do. Why is this, and is there any way to keep it from happening?

DR. LOIS: Smoking satisfies the oral needs. When a person stops smoking, she is withdrawing from a drug. The process is marked by irritability and nervousness, and some may be driven to nervous eating. The habits surrounding the lip and mouth movements are also satisfied by eating. They could just as well be satisfied by any chewing—even on a stick!

Yes, it takes willpower to stop smoking, but it takes even greater willpower not to turn to food as a comfort.

JUNE AND BARBARA: Ron Brown, a dietitian (now a physician) who used to work with us, told us that when he counseled diabetics about their diet he explained to them that Type I's need to be concerned mostly about the amount of carbohydrate they eat, and Type IIs about the amount of calories they eat. Do you agree with Ron on this, and could you elaborate?

**DR. LOIS:** I think Ron is right, and that's certainly an easily understandable way of explaining the main dietary guidelines. Appropriate dietary recommendations, in my opinion, must always be based on the patient's type of diabetes. The ideal diet for one type of diabetes may worsen control in another type.

I would like to go into more detail about the amount of carbohydrate that is ideal for each type of diabetes. There has been a good deal of controversy recently in scientific circles about high-carbohydrate diets. The question is, are they beneficial for persons with diabetes or not? I think we can shed some light on this issue.

First, let's mention that the goal of diet is to help you maintain normal blood sugars, so the ideal diet for you is the one that facilitates keeping your blood sugars within the normal range. With this in mind, we can divide diabetic people into three distinct categories.

## 1. INSULIN-DEPENDENT: COMPLETE PANCREATIC INSUFFICIENCY

If you are a Type I diabetic who produces no insulin of your own—we call this complete pancreatic insufficiency —then your problem is to calculate exactly how much insulin to inject to match the carbohydrate you eat. It is easier to match insulin with carbohydrate if you limit the total carbohydrate to 40 percent, most of which should be complex carbohydrate, high in fiber. Restricting carbohydrate to 40 percent will help you to avoid the rollercoaster effect: high blood glucose after you eat and low blood glucose about three hours later, when your insulin peaks.

## 2. INSULIN-REQUIRING: PARTIAL PANCREATIC INSUFFICIENCY

If you are insulin-requiring but your pancreas still secretes some insulin—partial pancreatic insufficiency—
then restricting carbohydrate may not help your blood
sugars. Since carbohydrate restriction decreases the
amount of insulin your own pancreas secretes, it is advisable for you to eat as much as 70 percent carbohydrate,
providing it is high in fiber. The higher percentage of
carbohydrate will prime your own insulin-producing
cells, and the fiber will slow down the conversion of
carbohydrate into simple sugars. The end result will be
blood sugars that are more consistently normal.

However, if you have difficulty matching your food to
insulin when you eat 70 percent carbohydrate, then you
are better off with 40 percent carbohydrate or maybe
even a little less.

## 3. NON–INSULIN-REQUIRING: OVERWEIGHT

If you are an overweight Type II diabetic, then you need
a restricted-calorie, restricted-carbohydrate diet. Again,
complex carbohydrate high in fiber is advised. The lowered amount of carbohydrate will allow the insulin receptors of your cells to function normally instead of
closing down, as they do when you overeat carbohydrate, stimulating your pancreas to overproduce insulin.

These dietary guidelines about the amount of carbohydrate to eat according to your type of diabetes are
controversial. We have no proof yet as to whether their

long-term effect will be beneficial. But in the interim, following these guidelines is the best choice.

As a final word I would add that diet prescription, in all cases, must be extremely individualized. You may prove to be an exception to any general dietary rule. Only your blood-sugar tests can tell you.

JUNE AND BARBARA: Before leaving carbohydrate amounts, could you explain the newer dietary system called "carbohydrate counting"? It has become popular of late, probably because of the increase in intensive therapy and the number of people using pumps. Our impression is that carbohydrate counting makes control for people on insulin much more precise and eliminates much of the guesswork of the past.

DR. LOIS: The peak past-meal blood-sugar response to a meal plan is directly related to the carbohydrate content of the meal. Fat is "free," so to speak. It does not raise your blood sugar or require insulin for its metabolism. (It does make us fat, however!) As for protein, only its amino acid (the building blocks of protein) converts to sugar and that takes about three hours, so it tends to buffer the leftover insulin taken for the meal. Thus, the only portion of the meal we need to cover with insulin is the carbohydrate.

The rule of thumb is 1.0 units of Regular insulin for every 10 grams of carbohydrate at lunch and dinner and 1.5 units of insulin for every 10 grams of carbohydrate at breakfast (to compensate for the dawn phenomenem). Then the dose of Regular is adjusted for the premeal blood sugar. If your blood sugar is normal, then only enough insulin to cover the carbohydrate is necessary. If it is low, then slightly less insulin is needed. If it is high, more insulin is needed. The sliding scale looks like this:

Blood sugar less than 70 = subtract 2 units
Blood sugar 71–100 = the 1.0 units for each 10 grams carbohydrate at lunch and dinner and 1.5 units at breakfast
Blood sugar 101–140 = add 2 units
Blood sugar over 140 = add 4 units

This "ratio" of insulin to carbohydrate is then adjusted according to the amount of carbohydrate you are going to eat. If a person starts dinner with a blood sugar of 90 mg/dl and eats 60 grams of carbohydrate and takes 6 units of Regular but goes up to a blood sugar of 300 after the meal, then the ratio is wrong. In that case the person needs one more unit for each 25 points above 300 to attain an after-meal blood sugar of about 150 (the highest normal after a meal). That means 6 more units of Regular were needed. Thus, the right dose of insulin would be 12 units for 60 grams of carbohydrate or 2 units per 10 grams of carbohydrate. Although most containers give the carbo content of the food on the label, I would recommend the following books: *Calories and Carbohydrates,* by Barbara Krauss, which lists 8,000 foods; *The Carbohydrate Gram Counter,* by Corinne Netzer, which lists 10,000 foods, and *The NutriBase Guide to Carbohydrates, Calories, and Fat* by Art Ulene, M.D., which lists a whopping 30,000 foods. With these, any food can easily be looked up and the right dose of insulin can be derived.

JUNE AND BARBARA: Perhaps the kinds of food that tempt us most are sweets in all their glorious forms. The human attraction to sweets goes way back to our earliest ancestors who, because we needed to have vitamin C in our diets, were programmed to like the sweet taste of fruit. Not only that, but as Dr. Lendon Smith writes in his foreword to the book *Sweet and Natural* (by Janet Warrington, Crossing Press, 1982), "Nature gave us taste buds to detect sweetness, and that sensory nerve goes right to the pleasure center of the brain." Until the new guidelines and latest research, people with diabetes were to thwart these natural tendencies and to deny themselves all forms of sweeteners except maybe a limited amount of artificial ones. Now, you still need to count carbohydrates and calories of course, but otherwise it's a brand new world.

Listen to these excerpts right out of the official American Diabetes Association Position Statement:

> "Scientific evidence has shown that the use of sucrose (sugar) as part of the meal plan does not impair blood glucose control in individuals with Type I or Type II diabetes. . . ."
>
> ". . . there is no reason to recommend that people avoid consumption of fruits and vegetables, in which fructose occurs naturally, or moderate consumption of fructose-sweetened foods." (Unless you have dyslipidemia.)
>
> "Nutritive sweeteners other than sucrose and fructose include corn sweeteners such as corn syrup, fruit juice or fruit juice concentrate, honey, molasses, dextrose (glucose), and maltose. There is no evidence that these sweeteners have any significant advantage or disadvantage over sucrose in terms of improvement in caloric content or glycemic response.
>
> "Sorbitol, mannitol, and xylitol are common sugar alcohols that produce a lower glycemic response than

> sucrose and other carbohydrates . . . There ap-
> pear no significant advantages of these sugar alco-
> hols over other nutritive sweeteners. Excessive
> amounts may, however, have a laxative effect."

And there you have it. Clear and simple. All caloric sweeteners are sisters under the skin.

Speaking of sweets, we've heard some research that may help explain why so many women are "chocoholics." Some scientists have discovered that eating chocolate produces the same chemical in the brain (phenylethylamine) as falling in love. That's why, when love has gone, people often go on chocolate binges to try to recapture that certain feeling. To make a nonfeminist generalization, that may be why there seem to be more women chocolate addicts than men. Women tend to be more susceptible to love. As Doris Lessing said, "Have you ever known a man who would interrupt his career for a love affair—and have you ever known a woman who wouldn't?"

Incidentally, there is good news for you chocolate lovers. It turns out that investigators have determined that the fat in chocolate isn't the artery-clogging type as we've all been led to believe. It seems that cocoa butter, the type of fat in chocolate, is converted in our livers to oleic acid before it can muck up our cholesterol metabolism. Oleic acid is a monounsaturate, just like that in olive or canola oil. Dark chocolate is the best choice, because the milk in milk chocolate does contain the bad-for-you-fat.

But enough of sweetness and love, let's get back to the basics of nutrition in the diabetic diet.

On to another nutritional question. Diabetic women often ask us about taking vitamin and mineral supplements. We have the feeling that since a diabetic woman may have a limited diet, she may not naturally get enough of the vitamins and minerals she needs. What is your opinion about this?

DR. LOIS: The recommended daily allowance (RDA) of calcium for a woman is 800 to 1,000 mg, in order to prevent brittle bones in old age. As it turns out, diabetes, when it is out of control, tends to erode bones faster than in persons without problems of hyperglycemia. Therefore, it is best to stay in good diabetic control and to eat more calcium, just in case.

Growing girls and pregnant or lactating women need even more calcium—at least 1,200 to 1,400 mg per day in order to prevent a negative balance of calcium at these times of increased need.

All other vitamins and minerals tend to be in normal balance in persons with diabetes, no matter what the level of control. The following is a list of RDAs for all women, diabetic or not:

| | |
|---|---|
| Vitamin A | 800.0 mg |
| Vitamin D | 5.0 mg |
| Vitamin E | 8.0 mg |
| Vitamin C | 60.0 mg |
| Thiamin | 1.0 mg |
| Riboflavin | 1.2 mg |
| Niacin | 13.0 mg |
| Vitamin $B_6$ | 2.0 mg |
| Folate (Folic Acid) | 400.0 mg |
| Vitamin $B_{12}$ | 3.0 mg |

(Although $B_{12}$ injections have been used as a treatment for diabetic nerve disease, there is no scientific proof that this works.)

| Phosphorus | 800.0 mg |
| Magnesium  | 300.0 mg |
| Iron       | 18.0 mg  |

(More iron may be needed if a woman has excessive periods or large blood losses with the delivery of her babies.)


A word of caution: Too much of a good thing may be poisonous. The vitamins and minerals that are toxic when taken in large doses include vitamin A, vitamin D, and iodine. Certain patients with iron-metabolism disease can get iron overload from too much iron. Thus, before embarking on a vitamin kick, it's best to consult a doctor about the right doses for you.


JUNE AND BARBARA: There's more and more information these days on the importance of fiber in the diet, especially with those recent reports reaffirming that it helps lower cholesterol, prevent cancer of the colon, and discourage the development of diabetes. It's awfully hard to get enough fiber in the diet—especially when you eat out a lot. What, therefore, is your opinion of using a fiber supplement such as Citrucel (sugar free) to make sure you have enough? We have one Type II woman who reports (anecdotal evidence!) that she's lowered her blood pressure, weight, and blood sugar simply by adding the fiber supplement.

Barbara has started drinking a glass of water with Citrucel in it morning and evening—especially when traveling. The reason she's something of a fanatic about it is that her father had a colostomy when she was in high school and she has hopes that fiber may win out over genes.

DR. LOIS: Although high-fiber diets have been shown to decrease the prevalence of bowel cancer and to improve some forms of colitis, plus decrease the levels of cholesterol in the bloodstream when more than 50 percent of the diet is composed of fiber, there is still no scientific proof that a high-fiber diet is specifically important for a person with diabetes. Because fiber increases gas formation and thus can be a nuisance, I would wait for more studies of diet for persons with diabetes before prescribing high-fiber diets to all my diabetic patients.

JUNE AND BARBARA: We know that the nutritional content of foods is vitally important. However, having written articles for such publications as *Gourmet*, *Bon Appétit*, and *Food and Wine*, we also feel that food is one of life's joys and not just a way of fueling the body and meeting the demands of insulin. As Dwight Eisenhower in his General days said, "Good food is more than sustenance, it's morale."

It's getting harder to keep your morale up with food these days, as Julia Child discovered. In a lecture we heard her complain that people are becoming afraid of food and eating it as if it were medicine when they should be thinking of it as a tasty treat and a pleasurable social experience. She maintains that with her attitude toward the importance of the enjoyment of foods she's a lot healthier than those who fret about every morsel they put in their mouths. "Look at me," she says with bright enthusiasm. "I'm eighty-five years old and I'm frisky as a . . . a . . . a *buffalo!*"

You, too, can be frisky as a buffalo and still keep your diabetes under control without succumbing to what Robert Ornstein, Ph.D., and David Sobel, M.D., authors of *Healthy Pleasures* call "Medical Terrorism."

They say—and we believe—that "worrying too much about anything, be it calories, salt . . . or cholesterol is bad for you."

The major problem with using food as medicine is that the prescription changes every month. We have an ongoing column in *The Diabetic Reader* called "The Fickle Finger of Food Facts." In this we point out how constantly changing the dictates of healthy dining are. For a while eating pasta is touted as a terrific way to lose weight: "Just be careful of the fat in the sauces; that's what puts on the pounds." Then almost as quickly as it takes pasta to reach the *al dente* stage, the finger swivels and Dr. Richard Heller of Mt. Sinai School of Medicine and co-author of *The Carbohydrate Addict's Diet* is telling us that no, for people with insulin resistance (the major problem of overweight Type II diabetics) carbohydrates, such as the highly touted pasta, cause you to overproduce insulin, which encourages the production of body fat, stimulates appetite and, over the long term, has serious health implications.

Butter? No, don't even look at the package. Margarine. *That's* the choice of the intelligent, health-conscious person. (Swivel.) Oh, oh, look out! The British medical journal *Lancet* reports: "Women who eat four or more teaspoons of margarine a day have a 50 percent greater risk of developing heart disease than women who eat margarine only once a month . . . Six or more teaspoons a day increases the risk to 70 percent."

Chocolate? It's a killer, and being a chocoholic is the next worse thing to being a heroin addict. (Swivel.) The wire services are humming with a love song for chocolate (see p. 198) But don't forget to watch out for the sugar in chocolate, or at least watch out for it until the ADA's new nutritional guidelines came out. (See the opening of this chapter.)

Every few months studies reveal that a certain vitamin or mineral supplement will practically make you immortal and then suddenly, (swivel) no, beware! Overuse of that product can cause serious, irreversible health problems.

What to do? What we do is to try to keep well informed on all the information about diet and health. The *New York Times* is our favorite source for the swivels and double reverse swivels of the Fickle Finger of Food Facts, but we never jump onto a food or food supplement bandwagon until it's circled the block a number of times. Often we're gratified to find that the things we really like, such as small amounts of butter instead of (ugh!) margarine, or olive oil (Extra Virgin, please!), or garlic (not only is it delicious, but it keeps vampires away) are actually considered the healthy route to take. We also try not to go overboard on *anything*, even those foods, drinks, and supplements that are the health flavor-of-the-month. That way when the inevitable swivel takes place, you won't be thrown into shock when you hear reports of how bad for you it is currently believed to be (before the next swivel reverses that opinion). If you don't follow any food dictate to its extreme, the best part is that you have a lot more variety in your diet, and this is the healthy and fun part of eating, anyway.

Speaking again of the fun part of eating, there's still another reason for having really delicious food: you need less of it to have a feeling of satisfaction, and this can help you control your weight. A well-known TV personality now scratching at the door of *le troisième âge* still looks lean and fit and terrific. Of course she does follow a good exercise program, but she also has a dining philosophy that helps. We once heard her say on a talk show that if she has, for example, a hamburger, she doesn't want it to be just a plain, average, run-of-the-mill hamburger that causes you to feel vaguely dissatisfied and hungry for more. No, she wants the definitive hamburger, the *perfect* hamburger, the hamburger-to-end-all-hamburgers, one that makes you feel you've had a wonderful experience and leaves you comforted and full of good feelings.

You've probably noticed this yourself. When you have something that's absolutely delicious, you may seem to get filled up very fast. For that reason, we always urge people with diabetes to become food snobs or, as they're called in Southern California, "foodies." After all, food is, as it has been said, "the most intimate consumer product." You put it into your body and make it a part of your body, so you should want it to be nothing but the freshest, the best-prepared, the most delightful. And, as a diabetic, since you must restrict how much you eat, it's particularly important that you shouldn't stint on how good it is any more than you do on how good *for* you it is.

The best way to ensure that you have the best of everything in the food department is to prepare it yourself. The lovely dishes you make yourself cost a fraction of the same thing in a restaurant. Cooking is a bad news/good news situation for a diabetic woman. The bad news is that you probably have to do most of the cooking for the family, and that takes a lot of time and effort in your busy schedule. The good news is that you *get* to do most of the cooking. The good news far outweighs the bad. When you do the cooking you can control what's served and make sure it's good for your diabetes control and health and good for your family. (Remember, the "diabetic diet" is nothing more than the healthy diet that everyone should be eating.) The more interesting and exotic dishes you learn to cook, the better understanding you have of what goes into these dishes so when you go out you're no longer thrown into confusion at the sight of a menu in a new restaurant. You're able to do what we think of as "dietary mainstreaming." You can eat anywhere anyone else can and enjoy yourself as much as they do and be totally relaxed about it.

But possibly the greatest advantage of learning to cook well and excitingly is the pleasure you'll derive from it. In 1995 the New York Public Library celebrated its one hundredth anniversary, and to commemorate the event they had a list of Books of the Century, "books that played defining roles in the past hundred years." One of the books on this exclusive list was *The Joy of Cooking*. And a joy it is if you cook with love and enthusiasm and the one-pointed attention to what you're doing that makes it a meditative and restoring experience. On top of that you and your family members and friends get to enjoy the fruits—and vegetables and viands—of your labor and live happily and healthily ever after.

But even with all this cheerleading for delightful diabetic dining, we do recognize there are restrictions involved and you'll sometimes wish you could eat in the relaxed, unthinking way nondiabetics do. Once June was talking to a twelve-year-old girl who had just been diagnosed as having diabetes, and, as is usually the case, had been stuffed full of diabetes information, with an emphasis on the dietary aspects. June, wanting to give her some hope for the future to hang on to, started telling her about all the possibilities for a cure, including beta cell transplants. The girl brightened up for the first time, and asked, "When that happens, will I be able to eat anything I want?"

This brought home to us again what a downer not being able to eat anything you want, whenever you want it is for most people. But when you come right down to it, this negative feeling is 80 percent a desire simply to feel free to eat anything you want. When you think you aren't allowed to eat something, it makes something that you would normally shun seem infinitely desirable.

This reminds us of a conversation we had with a woman who was one of the first persons to receive a pancreas transplant. After years of being a diabetic she suddenly *wasn't* one, and, boy, was she going to make up for lost time. We met her at breakfast during a diabetes conference. She was devouring pancakes that were swimming in maple syrup, and she told us that she had also been having a hot-fudge-sundae spree. She couldn't believe the miracle of being able to eat all the foods formerly forbidden to her.

We met her again a year later for lunch, and she was eating what appeared to be a perfect lunch for a diabetic. She had only a little fruit for dessert. What was going on? Had she turned diabetic again? Not at all. She told us that after a year of overindulgence in sweets and fats and anything else her formerly deprived heart and taste buds desired, she found that she had put on twenty pounds and felt perfectly rotten. She realized that this was no way to live, and she voluntarily went back to her former way of eating. In fact, she says she now follows a stricter regimen than she did as a diabetic, but she doesn't feel at all deprived because she's doing it by choice. As a result, she had slimmed back down and felt wonderful again.

So why don't you *pretend* that you've had a pancreatic transplant (who knows, you may have one before too long), and *pretend* that you've had your sweet-eating binge and gotten it out of your system, and *pretend* you're following your healthy eating plan because you want to look and feel good instead of just because you have to! You may just find that pretending—even more than wishing—will make it so.

# $\mathcal{E}$nvoi

## Not the Last Word

WHAT WE'VE GIVEN YOU HERE DEFINITELY ISN'T THE LAST word on the diabetic woman. There won't be a last word until the whole story of diabetes has a happy ending.

Diabetes is such a constantly changing field that even as we write this, new discoveries are being made that could alter the entire picture. For that reason, we encourage you to keep asking questions, and we'll keep trying to give you the answers. Write to us at Prana Publications, 5623 Matilija Ave., Van Nuys, CA, 91401 (1-800-735-7726). We'll forward your questions to Dr. Lois and publish her answers in *The Diabetic Reader*. Even if you don't have any questions, write to us to get on the mailing list for *The Diabetic Reader* so you can learn from the questions other women ask. If we receive a tremendous influx of questions, we'll update the book or even write a new one.

Keep in touch. We're all in this together, and if we join forces, as Susan B. Anthony said, "failure is impossible."

*207*

# Pregnancy
# Supplements

# $\mathscr{H}$ealthy, Happy Babies

## *A Private Consultation with Dr. Lois for Type I Women*

YOU WERE PROBABLY DIAGNOSED WITH DIABETES SEVERAL years ago, or perhaps you've just recently been diagnosed, but in either case, the diabetes came into your life before you became pregnant. My greatest hope is that you're reading this because you're now planning a pregnancy rather than just finding out that you're pregnant and saying, "Gee, I'm going to have a baby. What do I do now?" The reason I say this is that it's so much easier to plan to have a baby by first getting your blood sugars as close to normal as possible, rather than having to play catch-up by manipulating insulin, diet, and exercise to quickly normalize blood sugars so your baby does not experience any high blood sugars. So if we've got plenty of time because you're not pregnant, it certainly makes life easier for you and for your health care team.

Another reason why it's important to plan ahead and get your blood sugars in control is because the very first few precious moments of the baby's life, right after conception, are involved with the division of cells and the forming of organs. The organs of the body are formed by the second time you miss your period, meaning the first time you miss your period (about four weeks after your last period) the baby has already formed a heart. Six weeks after your last menstrual period, the baby is already forming nerve structures and a brain, and by eight weeks after your last menstrual period, which is missing your second period, the baby is completely formed. So during that time period it's most important that your blood sugars be absolutely normal, for any high blood sugars might interfere with the formation and growth and development of your baby's organs.

The most common problem an infant of a diabetic mother can develop is a heart defect or a hole in the heart. This happens when the mother's high blood sugar interferes with the closure of the membranes forming the heart. In addition, the tube that forms around the spinal cord becomes affected by high blood sugars and won't close, so neural tube defects are more common in infants of diabetic mothers if the blood sugars aren't normal before conception, or before the baby is actually formed. Also, babies can have trouble with the formation of their bowels and their brain. This list shows you how vitally important it is that your blood sugars be normal *before* pregnancy.

The risk of malformation and birth defects is as high as 25 percent for babies born of diabetic mothers who have high blood sugars. This means that even if blood sugars are high, there's still a 75 percent chance that nothing will happened to the baby at all. It's almost as though you need a genetic predisposition to have a child with a birth defect, and that predisposition is brought out by high blood sugars. The majority of women, no matter what their blood sugars are, will not have a birth-defective child. However a 25 percent chance is high enough that you shouldn't play Russian roulette, but rather you should get your blood sugars as near normal as possible before you conceive.

If you're already pregnant and perhaps even already past your eighth week of gestation, do not despair, for the 75 percent chance that your baby will be absolutely normal can be confirmed by tests of the baby. The first test is a sound-wave test or a sonogram. Sonography has advanced to the point where the heart, the brain and skull, and the spine can be visualized easily, but you'll have to wait until midway into your pregnancy to be able to see all these organs clearly and in detail. So you can be reassured things are going quite normally if you have patience and wait for the sonography tests.

Now, as you well know, it's not easy to normalize the blood sugars of a woman who has Type I diabetes. Blood sugars seem to have a mind of their own, as they ride the roller coaster of highs and lows, many of which seem to you to have no reason. I have a saying that "the wrong dose of insulin is the wrong dose of insulin," meaning that if your blood sugars aren't normal, your insulin dose is not right. You need to work with a health-care team to attain your ideal pattern of insulin doses. The team can help you bring your daily blood sugars into the normal range. Only the right insulin dose can do that for you. The easiest way to achieve good insulin adjustment is to go to the hospital for about a week for the kind of fine-tuning that you need. It may take four injections of insulin a day or an insulin infusion pump to get your blood sugars as near normal as possible. After discharge from the hospital you'll be on the telephone with the health care team every other day, perhaps daily even, and then it will slow down to once a week and once every couple of weeks until your blood sugars have stabilized and you're ready . . . are given permission to get pregnant.

Now we usually suggest that the starting insulin doses be about 0.6 times your weight in kilograms when you're not pregnant. This dose of insulin is the total twenty-four-hour insulin requirement. For a woman who weighs 60 kilograms, 0.6 times 60 kilograms is 36 units over twenty-four hours. In an NPH-and-Regular system, this is usually divided into three injections a day. The insulins are given so that your blood sugars are normal when you're not eating, and then each and every time you eat there's a perfect match of the insulin with the food.

To design a system like this means that you must take your NPH with Regular. The NPH is an intermediate-acting insulin that provides the basal need. The Regular is fast acting to cover the food you eat. Each dose of Regular insulin is adjusted according to your meal plan and your blood sugar at the moment. So you need a blood-sugar test before and one hour after the beginning of breakfast, lunch, and dinner, and then until the overnight blood sugars normalize, you'll need a bedtime and 3 A.M. check. As you see, signing up to have a baby is signing up for another job. Well, the only thing we're asking diabetic women to do is work harder . . . because the reward is magnificent. Normal blood sugars really do mean a normal baby.

Once the pregnancy has started, then we have to pay attention to each and every blood sugar so the organs form correctly. Thereafter growth and development are very much affected by high blood sugars. Sugar freely crosses the placenta. The baby reacts to the sugar that's in the mother's bloodstream. If the mother's bloodstream has a high sugar content, the baby will respond by secreting large doses of its own insulin. Remember, the baby does *not* have diabetes, but the end result of that increased insulin secretion will be that the baby grows too fat. All its energy goes into making fat and so it does not produce the amount of proteins, called enzymes, it needs to mature the brain and liver and lung function. If the baby is born prematurely, the baby will be very fat, will not be able to breathe, and will not have normal metabolism. In fact, the baby could die from having such high blood sugars because with its own metabolic balance being so off-kilter, it's incompatible with life. So you can see that even though it's hard work for nine months to have a healthy baby, it's well worth the energy invested. So roll up your sleeves, sign up for an intensive-care program, and really dig in and take good care of yourself moment to moment.

Once your blood sugars are in the normal range, then you can give yourself permission to get pregnant. We define normal as a fasting blood sugar of less than 90, and if you're not pregnant, a one-hour-after-beginning-the-meal blood sugar of 150. You also need a glycosylated hemoglobin or hemoglobin $A_{1C}$ test that is near normal. What is a glycosylated hemoglobin or hemoglobin $A_{1C}$? It's a wonderful test we have whereby we can grab a sample of your blood any time of day, regardless of meal plan or eating, test it, and find out how much of your hemoglobin is sugared. As it turns out, the hemoglobin, once it's sugared, stays sugared for the life span of the red blood cell. The hemoglobin is the pigment inside the red blood cell that is necessary to carry oxygen, so if it's floating around in your bloodstream for about 120 days, then the sugar content of that hemoglobin molecule will reflect the amount of sugar you've had in your bloodstream over approximately the last three to four months.

Normal, healthy people without diabetes have an average blood sugar of about 100, which means about 5 percent of their hemoglobin is sugared, so if the normal range is about 5 percent, we usually recommend that women with diabetes not get pregnant if their hemoglobin is sugared above 7 percent. Now these numbers will vary depending on the laboratory and depending on the test your physician orders. But what you really should suggest to yourself is that your hemoglobin $A_{1C}$ test should be in the normal range for the laboratory that your physician uses. If that is the case, then you have a positive signal to become pregnant.

Once you have this "permission" to become pregnant, you can try to conceive. What you should do is buy a basal body thermometer. This will allow you to chart your temperatures. Your temperature is about 96 in the morning before you get out of bed. And once you ovulate and the hormones surge, your temperature will go up to 97½ or even 98. At that exact moment when your temperature rises is when you're the most fertile. When you buy the basal body temperature thermometer, it comes with a wonderful package insert which teaches you how to use it and how to chart your temperatures. If, indeed, you've timed it perfectly, then it's very likely you will become pregnant. For the next two weeks, which is too early to do a blood test to find out if you're really pregnant, we have to pretend that you are. During this time your target blood sugars should be a before-meal blood sugar of less than 90 and a one-hour-after-the-meal of less than 120. Pregnant women have basically lower blood sugars than nonpregnant women, and therefore our target glucoses have to be lowered. Keeping your blood sugars in the target ranges means paying even more attention to detail. Perhaps at this moment you'll need either to come back into the hospital for readjustment or to increase the number of phone calls to your health-care team. Once again it's back to the weekly or every-other-day or even every-day phone call, if your blood sugars are not in the normal range. It does seem like a lot of work for both you and your health-care team, but it's very worth it to get on your way.

As the pregnancy progresses you will find your insulin requirements increase. This is a wonderful sign. It means the placenta is growing and making more hormones. Hormone action is against insulin and therefore the more hormones you have, the more insulin you'll need to take. The insulin requirement in the first twelve weeks of pregnancy is 0.7 units per kilogram of body weight per twenty-four hours. The hormone action and your weight both increase each week. From twelve to twenty-four weeks, the insulin requirement goes up to 0.8 times your weight in kilos. From twenty-four to thirty-two weeks it's 0.9 times your weight in kilos, and after thirty-two weeks—pregnancy is a total of 40 weeks—it's one unit per kilogram per twenty-four hours. So if you were a 60-kilogram woman before you became pregnant, your insulin requirement would be thirty-six units over twenty-four hours, and by the time you were ready to have the baby your insulin requirement would go up to sixty units over twenty-four hours.

The insulin adjustment doesn't happen overnight. It's every day one unit here, one unit there, two units here, two units there, as needed. Individual insulin doses are adjusted based on your blood sugar diary—two up and two down—and as the blood sugars rise a touch here, a touch there. The insulin dosages must be adjusted so baby never sees a bad blood sugar. This kind of skill will be useful to you for the rest of your diabetic life. Learning to adjust insulin for diet, exercise, and stress is a wonderful fund of knowledge that will help you forever, and therefore it's well worth the effort not only to have a healthy baby, but really to plan the rest of your life.

As your pregnancy is growing and you're charting ev-

ery day, of course, seeing your increased insulin requirements—a good sign—you'll probably be scheduled for a
sonogram in the middle of your pregnancy. This is the
point in your pregnancy when the physicians can see
your baby's organs and bone structure, can count the
vertebrae going down the baby's back, can see that the
baby has ten fingers and ten toes. At this point, the obstetrician may be able to tell whether or not you have a
boy or a girl. This can be a very reassuring time, because
the doctor can actually verify that your baby is just fine.
In addition, the obstetrician can tell you whether your
baby's growing too quickly. Overgrowth of the infant
often means that your blood sugars are not in the normal
range.

Besides checking your blood sugar diary, your physician should be measuring your hemoglobin $A_{1C}$ every
month. Your goal is to have an $A_{1C}$ in the low normal
range, because blood sugars of normal pregnant women
are at the rock-bottom lowest of normal and even
slightly below the normal range. Ideally, laboratories
would have a pregnant range but many laboratories have
not developed such ranges. So target yourself to be on
the low range of normal and then you'll be doing super.
In our laboratories we do have a pregnancy range. Our
nonpregnant range is from 4.9 to 6.1 percent. Our pregnant women have to be 4.5 to 5.0 percent. If you are 5.0
or under, your baby really will be growing normally, for
it's only the sugar that's the problem with the infant of
the diabetic mother.

Incidentally, $A_{1C}$ is affected by temperature, humidity,
and technical expertise. Thus, the test can vary from
month to month with the weather and the changeover of
technical staff. The easiest way to use a local lab for the
$A_{1C}$ is to send the blood to the lab with a normal control.
The best control would be a pregnant woman without

diabetes who is in the same week of gestation. Short of such an ideal control, a fit, lean, athletic husband will do. (Athletes tend to have lower mean blood-glucose levels than nonathletes.) I then demand that the pregnant diabetic woman's $A_{1C}$ be lower than her husband's before I would deem her to be in good control.

Besides the baby, we also have to be concerned about certain of the mother's problems resulting from diabetes. If you started this pregnancy with long-standing diabetes, it may be that your eyes and kidneys have a touch of diabetic complications. Therefore on the team you need an ophthalmologist looking at your eyes every month if you have any hint of retinopathy or eye disease at the back of your eye. Even if you have no retinopathy, your ophthalmologist should examine you as soon as you're pregnant and at the end of pregnancy to make sure there have been no changes due to the stresses of pregnancy.

In addition, you need kidney function tests, with a twenty-four-hour collection of every drop of urine paired with a blood test called a creatinine clearance. It's very important to document how much protein you may be spilling throughout your pregnancy, for women with diabetes have a tendency to have an increased risk of another disease during pregnancy called toxemia. Toxemia is a name given to a condition developed by women who develop hypertension or high blood pressure during pregnancy. It's a separate disease with separate risks for the baby, and therefore you should be collecting twenty-four-hour urine specimens (every drop for twenty-four hours) during the first, second, and third trimesters, documenting how much protein you spill, and having your blood pressure measured at every office visit. Your health-care team knows the risk factors, knows the points along the way where they need to intervene. High blood pressure is actually a more severe danger for your baby than blood sugar, so it must be watched very carefully. Because you have diabetes, you are at a higher risk for high blood pressure during pregnancy.

We also have to ask you to make sure your obstetrician remembers to check your urine for infection. Diabetic women have an increased risk for a urinary tract infection during pregnancy, so if your obstetrician sort of forgets, just remind him or her that you need your urine checked frequently to make sure that you don't have a urinary infection.

Now, back to what else you should monitor. Many obstetricians feel that you should also monitor ketones. This is true if your blood sugar ever gets above a certain target level, and most obstetricians claim that above 200 is the number indicating a need to measure urine for ketones. Ketones confer a separate risk for the unborn child. They interfere with intelligence. Therefore, we don't want you to spill any ketones whatsoever. If you see a touch of ketones, very quickly you need your insulins adjusted so that never happens again. Your obstetrician will guide you in terms of how often and when to measure your urine for ketones. But if your blood sugars are always in the normal range or the near-normal range, then you don't have to worry about ketones. They usually only develop when the diabetes is out of control.

Besides measuring blood sugars and adjusting insulin, a major part of your success depends on learning how to match the insulin with food. We suggest that your health-care team include an expert in nutrition in pregnancy so that you get the adequate amount of vitamins and minerals and an understanding of how to match insulin with food so precisely that your blood sugars will not go high. This could well be your most difficult task.

Meal planning is a real challenge during pregnancy. Don't be surprised if your physician can't help you at all with diet. Many of us were not taught a thing about diet and nutrition at medical school, and we're very dependent on our expert on the team, the dietitian. She/he really is skilled at translating formulas and menus and meal plans into what can be reality for you. Spend a lot of time with her/him and make sure that you and your husband understand the best possible way to normalize blood sugar before you leave the dietitian's office. A dietitian is a wonderful resource, and you shouldn't hesitate to call if you have questions even as you open your cookbook.

The rule of thumb is that you must stay away from simple sugars. A simple sugar eaten immediately after your insulin injection will zing into your bloodstream and will peak well before the insulin action begins. The best strategy is to have a lag time. The lag time should vary based on your blood-sugar reading before the meal. For instance, if you're low before the meal, which we define in pregnancy to be less than 60, you could inject and eat right away. In this case, some of your meal plan is being used to treat your hypoglycemia. You can even take a little less insulin if your blood sugar is less than 60, for that food portion that corrects the hypoglycemia is subtracted from the meal and then you're left with a smaller meal and you need less insulin.

If your blood sugar's between 60 and 90, which is a normal premeal blood sugar, even for a woman who does not have diabetes, you just need to take enough insulin to cover the meal plan. This insulin needs time to get out from under the skin into the bloodstream, and that takes about thirty minutes. Eat your protein and your fat first and save the carbohydrates until the tail end of the meal, because insulin, although it has its onset at thirty minutes, doesn't peak until an hour and a half after it's injected. You want the punch power of the insulin to cover your carbohydrates. The proteins and fats do not impact on your blood sugar immediately.

If your blood sugar's between 90 and 110, you'll need one or two extra units of insulin in addition to your usual dose. On the other hand, if you were low, you'd subtract a unit or two. The insulin dosage works on a sliding scale. If you're superhigh, which we define as anything above 120, take two to four extra units, depending on how insulin resistant you are. Of course, the lag time between the injection and eating will be longer if your blood sugar's very high, because you'll need time for the insulin to bring the blood sugar down to normal before you can eat your meal. If you are high, wait until you're down to 150 and then start eating immediately. (We have to keep you from crashing when the insulin starts working strongly.)

Now it may be that you wake up high and take your normal breakfast insulin plus two to four units extra, but your blood sugar never comes down to 150, so you don't get to eat breakfast. In this case, at lunchtime, you should take another extra dose of insulin with your lunch injection and then wait until you're below 150. You'll be able to eat lunch but since you may have gone a long time without eating, as soon as your blood sugar's 150, gobble up the food you've prepared. This is a gentle way to bring down the blood sugar without overdosing yourself with large doses of insulin in one package. Large doses can cause a later crash.

The next advice for this meal plan is not to eat any carbohydrates for breakfast and certainly not to drink fruit juices at breakfast. It's much easier to take a low dose of Regular insulin at breakfast, because you don't have much carbo in the meal plan and therefore you won't crash at midmorning from the peak of a high dose of Regular insulin. (Regular hits you an hour and a half to two hours later.) Regular doesn't cover the simple or complex sugars in your meal plan quickly enough. Once we have a quicker insulin (called lyspro and now being developed), we can change all these rules, but until it's available we need to ask you to minimize the amount of carbohydrate in breakfast.

So what does breakfast look like if you can't have the classic American breakfast—juice, toast, cereal, jam, waffles—all those delicious-sounding traditional foods that absolutely have to be avoided during pregnancy? The best meal plan for breakfast actually is a pure protein-fat breakfast—fat does not convert to glucose and therefore is there for calories for nutrition for you and your baby. Don't worry about heart disease. Your estrogen levels, the hormones coming from your placenta, are high enough so that at the moment you're not at risk for any heart disease due to the increased cholesterol you might be ingesting, so enjoy at least your fats in your meal plan, and use them to provide the extra calories that you won't be allowed to eat in extra carbohydrates.

The best meal for breakfast would be an egg omelet with last night's meat, fish, chicken, or cheeses all put into it. Or you could have cottage cheese or hard cheeses or yogurts. The plain nonfat yogurts are marvelous, but don't pick yogurts with the jellies in it or the ones that are sweetened. Pick plain yogurts, and then you can throw in a little bit of chopped apple. I'll allow you an apple at breakfast because apples do have fiber, which will minimize the amount of quickly absorbed sugar, but no apple juice. In fact the only juice you're allowed at breakfast is tomato juice—no orange or grapefruit juice.

You can also have vegetables and lemons or lemon juice and tomatoes if that's what you'd like. The amount of calories in this kind of breakfast will not have an impact on your blood sugar, but they will make you fat. Ask your dietitian to help plan how many calories you should eat. Your total twenty-four-hour caloric requirement is calculated based on your body weight. You need thirty calories per kilogram of weight. If you take your weight in kilograms and multiply it by 30, you'll come out to the amount of calories you need both for yourself and your unborn child. The calories need to be distributed so that fewer than 40 percent are carbohydrates, with a caveat that breakfast have almost no starch whatsoever.

Now although milk does contain sugars in the form of lactose or milk sugar, you need the calcium it provides. I am restricting the pure starches such as toast, cereal, potatoes, rice, and pasta throughout your meal plan to give you plenty of room to enjoy milk. Also, you can use milk to treat hypoglycemia or drink an extra glass here or there when you're slightly low.

At midmorning, if you're hungry, apples and cheese are a wonderful snack to prevent what's called starvation ketosis, which means that if you go too long without eating your body will burn its own fat and produce ketones. And as we've pointed out, we want to minimize the ketones in your blood. A midmorning snack is also worthwhile so that you won't be so hungry at lunch that you'll have trouble not eating out the whole refrigerator.

Lunch and dinner look about the same: they're basically as much protein (fish, meat, poultry, eggs, cheese) as you want, all the vegetables you can eat, and lots of salad. Be careful with the salad dressing, though. Read the labels to make sure that you're not getting any hidden sugars. It's probably best to make your own oil and vinegar salad dressings with spices. Spices are free; they don't have sugar in them. If you don't have trouble with your blood pressure, you're welcome to use as much salt

as your palate desires. You can have corn or beans, because they're complex starches with lots of fiber, but
once again I've restricted the pure starches: breads, rice,
potatoes, pasta.

You can have a snack in the afternoon, too. Here we
suggest apples and cheese again. At bedtime you can
have another snack, one with a mixture of protein, fat,
and a little bit of carbohydrate. This provides a buffer
for the 3 A.M. low that may occur if your overnight insulins are a little too strong for you. It's nice to go to bed
with a tummy full of food that's not so quickly absorbed
that it's gone within an hour. Our favorite bedtime snack
is ice cream, believe it or not. About a Dixie cup's worth
will provide enough sugar, protein, and fat to keep your
sugars normal until 3 A.M. and still make it possible for
your physician to give you enough long-acting insulin to
lower your wake-up blood sugar.

I'm sorry to interrupt your sleep, but I do ask that you
get up at 3 o'clock in the morning and measure your
blood sugar. You do this to make sure you will come up
with a good fasting blood sugar. If your blood sugar is
slightly high at 3 o'clock, you need a little more insulin
at that hour because of the dawn phenomenon (the rising of the blood sugar that comes with the rising of the
sun). If your sugar's slightly high at 3 A.M., it will be
much higher at 7 A.M. So a test at 3 A.M. gives you the
opportunity, if your blood sugar is high, to take a little
extra Regular so that the next morning you'll have a
normal blood sugar. On the other hand, if your blood
sugar is low, you can treat that and fix it for the following morning by lowering your bedtime NPH. When
you wake up with a normal blood sugar, it's incredible
how beautifully the day goes. When you wake up with a
high blood sugar, you spend the whole day trying to get
out of the mess. Therefore, it's worth taking a few min-

utes in the middle of the night to make sure tomorrow goes smoothly.

As the pregnancy progresses, your doctor will increase tests of the baby to make sure he/she is healthy. These tests will include not only more sonograms but also more opportunities to weigh and measure, look at the amount of amniotic fluid, look at cardiac function, look at what's called a biophysical profile, and trying to see if the baby is moving at a right frequency and stretching and doing breathing exercises. All these tests are done to reassure you and the obstetrician that things are going just fine.

If your blood sugars are absolutely normal and you have no complications such as high blood pressure, the watchful waiting will continue. The doctor wants the baby to be delivered as close to the normal due date as possible. If, however, your physician feels that the baby may be at risk, that some things have not gone as beautifully as he or she had wished, then the baby may have to be delivered early. In this case, there will need to be a baby lung test, which your obstetrician will do for you. In this test a bit of amniotic fluid is taken to see whether the baby is ready to breathe, for the biggest risk with a premature infant is that the baby can't quite breathe yet and needs to be put on a respirator.

You know that a baby can breathe when the lungs open up and expand and remain open with a soapsuds-like material called surfactant. The obstetrician will be looking for surfactant that's in the amniotic fluid, because as the baby is doing exercises, pretending to breathe, it will breathe in and out the amniotic fluid. As the amniotic fluid goes into the baby's lungs, it washes out some of these "soapsuds," and when this material appears in the amniotic fluid, it means the baby's ready to breathe.

Once positive pulmonary function has been documented, then it's safe to deliver the baby as soon as possible. Obstetricians will tell you that if your baby's over five pounds, generally he or she will do just fine. You can actually quiz your obstetrician and ask him or her what the indications for delivery are, what would be best for the infant, does the baby get a lung test, whether you can have a trial labor. You should also ask the doctor if he/she thinks it'd be okay for you to try to see if you can push the baby out, because if your blood sugars have been normal the baby won't be too big for a vaginal delivery. One of the complications of a very overweight baby is that it can get injured as it's being pushed through the birth canal; so if the baby's just the right size, you do have an opportunity to try to deliver vaginally.

If everything's a go and your obstetrician says yes, you can have a trial labor. Once the first contraction comes, you need to cut your doses of insulin way down. And, in fact, the rule of thumb is that when the first contraction comes and you're at home, don't take any more insulin and don't eat anything more but go immediately to the hospital. It may be, though, that your obstetrician will tell you to stay home and wait until the contractions come every two to five minutes. If that's the case and you're told not to eat anything, it really is okay to suck on popsicles, because the sugar will get into your bloodstream to keep your blood sugar up as you're exercising with the contractions, which burn your sugar. You suck on these popsicles (not the sugar-free but the sugar-full popsicles) because you'll be burning a lot of energy and you'll need a little sugar to keep on going.

The anesthesiologist, who is on standby to put you to sleep if you need a cesarean section, doesn't want you to have anything to eat for hours. It's not cheating to eat a popsicle, though, because the sugars are very quickly absorbed through the lining of your mouth and stomach. Essentially your stomach will remain empty even if you're eating popsicles. So stock up on your favorite flavor of popsicles for that moment when you go into labor and your sugar drifts a little low and your obstetrician says to stay home and wait till the contractions come more frequently. The exercise of labor really does lower the blood sugar, so don't be surprised if you get to eat a popsicle every hour to keep your blood sugar between 60 and 120, which is a perfect place to be while you're having labor.

As soon as the baby's out, your blood sugars will drop quite quickly, because as we discussed, the increasing insulin requirement, which goes up from the time before you're pregnant to the end of pregnancy almost 40 to 50 percent, drops immediately as soon as the placenta's delivered—so this is a time when we've actually got an opportunity to pig out and not worry about our blood sugars. Also, you may find out that you don't even need to take insulin for the first forty-eight hours. We call this period the "honeymoon." It's a time when the leftover insulins are getting out of your bloodstream. There's no need for extra insulin because you're no longer having to fight the stress of the hormones from the placenta. This is a period of time when you could easily have an insulin reaction. It's almost best to err on the lower side of insulin doses than the higher side.

What we usually do is recalculate the insulin doses as though you weren't pregnant at all, as now you no longer are! We put into the equation 0.6 times your weight in kilos and then we actually don't give the bedtime dose of insulin, allowing you to drift up a little bit and get some room to breathe. This adjustment of insulin does call for an expert. It needs to be individualized as every woman is different after her baby's born, but the rule of thumb is you'll need much less insulin. If it seems to you that the doctors haven't decreased your doses of insulin from the time before you went into labor, complain. Say that you're not pregnant, you need much less insulin, and in fact insulin requirements will clearly be documented by doing frequent blood sugars.

And, yes, we want you to breast-feed. Breast-feeding is not only a wonderful way to bond with your baby, but also there's some literature that claims that breast-fed babies of Type I women have a decreased risk of getting diabetes. I know that sounds weird, but actually it has to do with the milk the baby can absorb. Cow's milk may create an allergy in the infant if the baby has the right genetic predisposition, and the baby's allergy will attack not only the milk molecule but also the baby's pancreas. It's a very curious phenomenon. If it's true, however, we don't want the baby ever to see cow's milk, because the allergy is the strongest against cow's milk and doesn't occur against human milk. If you can continue to breast-feed for at least three to six months, the chances are fewer that your baby will develop Type I diabetes. But don't worry: The risk of your baby developing Type I diabetes is only 2 percent of all of your children, so if you have 100 children, yes, two of them are likely have diabetes.

During breast-feeding you must maintain normal blood sugars, because if your sugar's above 120 the extra sugar in your bloodstream will spill into the milk and the milk will be too sweet. This sweetness gets the baby to like sugar and, who knows, this may be how you create sugar junkies. Also with the extra calories from the sugar, your baby will be overnourished. After all, your baby was born at just the right size and shouldn't start getting too fat now, increasing the number of fat cells and making it easier to gain and harder to lose weight in later life. In addition, if you breast-feed until your baby has his or her first teeth, the extra sugar will increase the risk of dental caries. For all sorts of reasons, then, it's best to keep your blood sugar as near normal as possible while you're breast-feeding, but please be careful with your overnight insulin doses. When your baby drinks your milk, he or she is pulling from you milk sugar, the lactose in your milk. The milk sugar pulled from you will decrease your insulin requirements, specifically overnight when you are not eating.

So now you and your husband have a very happy, healthy baby. Congratulations! The fruits of your labor have been well worth the effort. Please take good care of yourself and stay in touch with your health-care team, for now you've just become a postpregnant person and need to learn how to keep your blood sugars normal, even when you're not having a baby.

# $\mathcal{H}$ealthy, Happy Babies

## *A Private Consultation with Dr. Lois for Women with Gestational Diabetes*

GESTATIONAL DIABETES, AS YOU MUST ALREADY HAVE BEEN told when you received the diagnosis, is diabetes that appears during pregnancy. At this point I know that you're probably upset, concerned and wondering "Why me?" After all, as soon as you found out that you were pregnant, or even before you were pregnant, you took the best possible care of yourself. You ate the right foods, you stayed away from everything your physician told you to avoid. Why then did this diabetes thing happen to you? You mustn't feel guilty. Getting gestational diabetes is not your fault. The problem is that diabetes is in your gene structure; you inherited a tendency toward diabetes. (If you're not careful, diabetes may recur as you age, but we'll talk about trying to prevent this later.) You developed gestational diabetes because your genetic predisposition precipitated the high blood sugars.

Pregnancy, of course, is a time in your life when you're gaining weight, but you're supposed to! Be that as it may, your body doesn't know the reason why you're gaining weight. It only knows that it can't keep up with the ever increasing insulin requirement. Insulin, the hormone that helps the body cells take up sugar from the blood, is made by your pancreas. Your pancreas is an organ situated behind your stomach, and it secretes insulin perfectly matched for the food that comes into your stomach. When you outgrow the size of your pancreas, of course your insulin needs increase but your pancreas can't make enough insulin to keep up with these additional needs. Therefore, your blood sugar goes up. Thus in the middle of your pregnancy, right at about week twenty of gestation, the diagnosis of gestational diabetes is made.

The diagnosis is made from a test in which you take a sugar drink. Because when you're not eating anything your blood sugar may be perfectly fine, the test is taken in a fasting state. Given the sugar challenge of the drink, your pancreas may not able to secrete enough insulin to take care of you and the unborn child, so the blood sugars measured after the drink are most important for the diagnosis. If indeed your blood sugars are up, the obvious treatment is to restrict sugars so that your pancreas doesn't have to overwork.

Gestational diabetes technically means diabetes that occurs only during pregnancy or gestation. In 80 to 90 percent of all women who have gestational diabetes, the diabetes goes away completely as soon as the baby is born. However, gestational diabetes will recur during each subsequent pregnancy if the amount of weight loss is not significant between pregnancies. You have an opportunity after this baby has been born to go on a weight-loss program that may prevent subsequent diabetes in the future. But for now we have to treat you as though you do have a serious disease.

This disease is the most common medical problem

affecting pregnant women in the United States. About fifty thousand women a year are diagnosed with gestational diabetes. It tends to happen to women of certain ethnic backgrounds. For instance, in some national groups such as Viennese (from Austria) and people from Newcastle, England there is a very low prevalence of diabetes in the gene structures, while in other groups such as Native Americans, Mexican Americans, and African Americans there is a very high prevalence. The prime example of a group with high incidence of diabetes is the Pima Indians. In that population 50 percent of all persons in the tribe have a tendency toward diabetes mellitus! So you can see that as far as diabetes is concerned, you're sort of a victim of your gene structure.

Now what happens if we don't treat your gestational diabetes, or you didn't get the diagnosis because your doctor didn't give you the sugar drink? Well, unfortunately, your baby would be the one to suffer. If your diabetes is mild you don't feel a thing, but still your sugars are high enough to prevent normal growth and development in the baby. The sugar freely crosses the placenta, and the baby, who does not have diabetes, responds appropriately to the hyperglycemic stimulus of the high blood-sugar levels coming from you by secreting a lot of insulin. Over time, insulin plus sugar cause obesity. Therefore, the baby grows very fat from this overnutrition at the expense of using energy to develop the lungs, brain, and liver normally. This overweight baby will also be very difficult to deliver through the birth canal. In addition, because the baby is premature in every other way, it will have difficulty breathing and functioning once it's born. Severe high blood sugars untreated could subsequently even cause the death of the baby. But it's easy with proper treatment to make your blood sugars normal; then your baby won't know that you have diabetes and will be absolutely normal. Our task today is to teach you to take care of yourself now that you have the diagnosis of gestational diabetes, and to be certain that you know exactly the blood sugars your baby is experiencing.

The diagnosis of gestational diabetes should be made at exactly at the moment when you develop the diabetes. That's the idea of giving you the sugar drink, not at the beginning, but in the middle of your pregnancy. We have to wait for a sufficient amount of physical stress to bring out all your diabetic tendencies. But don't worry, the baby isn't sick yet from your high blood sugars. In fact, an interesting test for you to ask your doctor to order is one called glycosylated hemoglobin or hemo-globin $A_{1C}$. This test reflects your average blood-sugar levels over a period of approximately 120 days. If your glycosylated hemoglobin level is normal, then you know that your sugars were normal in the past so that there was no risk to your baby. But now you have received the diagnosis of high blood sugar. If we immediately start treating those blood sugars, your baby really won't think you have diabetes at all. In addition, this hemoglobin $A_{1C}$ test is important because it allows us to compare you to you. Each and every month from now on you should have that test repeated, for if subsequent tests equal to-day's results or indeed if you get an even lower result, you know that what you're doing with your treatment plan is absolutely perfect.

So what's so bad about a big baby? Well, I think it's worth working on trying to keep you as healthy as possi-ble and your baby as healthy as possible. Yes, you could have a cesarean section so the baby could be taken from you without any birth trauma whatsoever, but it would be nice to keep the baby at a normal weight so you could have a normal vaginal delivery without hurting you or the baby. In addition, if the baby is very sick he or she would need intensive care for about two to ten days, depending on the degree of illness. Wouldn't it be nice to have your baby immediately in the recovery room and in your room so that the two of you could go home together?

It's as simple as that. Yes, doctors know how to treat the baby if the baby is suffering from your high blood sugars, but wouldn't it be wonderful to have a healthy baby who doesn't have any problem whatsoever for the doctors to treat? Since of course that's what we want, we have to roll up our sleeves now and begin to do a lot of work.

The first thing you have to realize is that the baby experiences every blood sugar in your bloodstream, no matter what time of day or night it is. So in order to know whether or not our treatment plan is working, you have to learn how to measure your own blood sugar. This is done by a simple kit that allows you to prick your own finger with a very fine needle, squeeze up a drop of blood, put it on a reagent strip (which is a stick that comes in a container), wait the appropriate amount of time, and then wait to see if the stick changes color. Either you can read the stick visually and match it to a color chart on the side of the bottle, or you can rent or buy a testing machine that allows you to put the stick inside the machine and have the machine read the blood sugar accurately. In either case we feel the best possible therapy is to keep the wake-up before-breakfast blood sugar (called a "fasting blood sugar") below 90 milligrams per deciliter and the highest blood sugar, which is one hour after beginning a meal, less than 120 milligrams per deciliter. These target glucose levels have been shown to be the upper limits of normal; and if the blood sugars are less than 90 before a meal and no higher than 120 one hour after a meal, your baby will be absolutely normal. You should ask your physician to refer you to a nurse educator or a pharmacist to teach you these tools and techniques so you can get accurate results from your test.

Once you've learned how to measure your blood sugar accurately, you need to know how to chart the results properly, because the best way to help you with your blood-sugar control is to look at your data records and make decisions based on you and your lifestyle. You need to chart not only your blood sugars, but also what foods you've eaten, what emotions, stresses, or illnesses have been in your life, and what kind of exercising you've been doing. With this information, decisions can be made with the total picture in front of the health-care provider.

So now you've learned how to check your blood sugar and how to chart your blood sugars, food, and activities. Now you need to learn about the mainstay of your therapy: diet. After all, if you don't put the sugar into your bloodstream, the sugar won't get into the baby's bloodstream. You have a good opportunity to maintain your blood sugars in the normal range if on your glucose-tolerance test your fasting blood sugar was below 90. If it was above 90 but less than 100, the chances are also good that your blood sugars will be normal. If your blood sugar is less than 90, once again there is no problem with maintaining your blood sugars with diet alone. You just have to restrict certain foods in your meal plan. Therefore, closer contact with your health-care team needs to be made as you try on the diet for size and see if it fits.

If your fasting blood sugar on your glucose-tolerance test is much above 100, then one week of dietary trial is worthwhile. If you cannot maintain your target blood sugars below a fasting level of 90 and a one-hour-after-the-meal level of less than 120, it's an absolute indication for you to start taking some more insulin, because your body is not making enough for you to take care of you.

So let's talk about the diet. You should be given a nutritious diet with sufficient calories to maintain your weight—not to lose or gain weight, but just weight maintenance calories. And the composition of that diet should be such that it never makes your blood sugars go up much above the baseline blood sugar you have when you wake up. In order to do this, we have to restrict sugars and carbohydrates. You may be asking, "What is a carbohydrate?" Carbohydrates are the form of nutrients you eat that are chains of sugars. Because your body breaks them down into simple sugars in your bloodstream, we have to minimize the carbohydrates as well as the simple sugars.

Let's start with the easy things to avoid, those that make a big impact on raising your blood sugar. Those are the simple sugars such as glucose, fructose, sucrose, table sugar, and fruit sugars. You can read food labels, and if there is an "ose" at the end of the name, it means this ingredient is a simple sugar. The foods to be avoided are essentially cookies, candies, cakes, sodas with sugars in them, and of course ice creams with sugars and all the other sweet things that seem so wonderful. Essentially, for the rest of your pregnancy, I want you to feel as though you're allergic to these foods, as though if you touch them you'll turn into one big boil. It is much easier to avoid these foods completely than to have the stress and concern that eating some of them might make your blood sugars go up out of the normal range.

The starches or complex carbohydrates need to be minimized but not 100 percent avoided. We handle these judiciously. A complex carbohydrate is a starch that the body breaks down into simple sugars. Examples of starches, or complex carbohydrates, are: breads, rice, pasta, potatoes, cereals, bagels, etc. But you understand, of course, that this list represents only a portion of the starchy foods that will eventually become sugars in your bloodstream.

A meal plan should be devised for you that has less than 40 percent of its total content composed of carbohydrates. The main caveat of this meal plan is that the breakfast meal be very small and almost devoid of starch, because your pancreas is the most sluggish in the morning since it's fighting a lot of stress just by your waking up in the morning, and stress-related production of hormones makes your own insulin weaker. Your plan for breakfast, therefore, should consist of mostly protein because your pregnancy causes very high hormone levels. These hormones, specifically estrogen, will protect you against heart disease, so for this one moment in your life it's wonderful to be able to tell you that you don't have to worry about cholesterol. Breakfast can have quite a bit of fat in it because fat does not become sugar—but, remember, it can't have any starch. Here's an example of a breakfast that is completely devoid of carbohydrates. It consists of an egg omelet, which could be prepared with the dinner meat, fish, or cheese of the night before. This meal is 100 percent protein and fat. It has about 400 calories, so you won't be hungry, but it won't make your blood sugar go up. The only fruit juice you're allowed is tomato juice. Yes, tomatoes are fruit, but even so, you are allowed tomato juice. Every other form of fruit juice is absolutely forbidden. The sugars in juice immediately get into your bloodstream; it's the wrong thing for breakfast, when your pancreas is so sluggish. So please don't drink fruit juice no matter how much you want to.

As far as fruits are concerned, you'll be allowed certain fruits later on in the day once your pancreas has awakened. Examples of these fruits are lemons, limes, and I would particularly recommend that you have apples. Apples are very high in fiber, and most of the sugars in them will not be absorbed. Do not, of course, drink apple juice because it breaks down the fibers and becomes pure sugar juice. So please, at the moment, watch your fruits. We'll try them on for size, and when you come back for a checkup we can see whether or not your blood sugars have maintained a normal range and you're ready for an increase in carbohydrates and fruits; and we can see where you have room for the fruits you've been dying for—perhaps in an afternoon snack. But that's at the next visit; it's not now. Now is the time when you need to know whether or not you can tolerate certain foods and, therefore, whether or not you really need insulin therapy.

After this breakfast, by midmorning you may become very hungry. Fortunately, midmorning is far enough away from the wake-up hormones so that you will be able to have some apples and cheese at 10:30. At noon you may have your lunch, which is mostly protein and fat—specifically fish, meat, chicken, turkey, all types of poultry, of course, cheeses, and all the salads in the world. Be careful of salad dressings, though. Read the labels carefully and watch out for those simple sugars that many of them contain. It might be safer just to make your own oil-and-vinegar dressing (without sugar, of course). You may use all the herbs and spices you want; there is no sugar in them. If you don't have a problem with your blood pressure, you may also put as much salt on your food as you want. But be careful with those starches.

At lunch I'd like you to begin with having the equivalent of one slice of bread. You may have an alternative portion of rice, but only eat as much rice as would be equal in proportion to the slice of bread. You may have a potato, but again only equal to one slice of bread. We call it one bread exchange, or the equivalent of a slice of bread you are allowed at lunch. For dessert you may have an apple, which provides a little bit more carbohydrate. But these sugars won't get into your blood stream, so don't worry. Please have as much milk at lunch and dinner as you want. I have restricted your starches so you can tolerate the lactose or milk sugar in milk. I want you to get enough calcium, so at the moment we will not restrict your milk. What we will do is look at your blood sugars, and if there is a problem we might ask you to adjust the amount of milk you drink; but at the moment I would rather steal from the bread exchanges than rob you of such an important food as milk.

In the afternoon if you're hungry you can have some more apples and cheese or leftover protein from your lunch. Dinner should look very much like lunch. The total number of calories you should be eating if, according to your physician, you're at about the right weight, ought to be a total of 30 calories per kilogram of your current weight. If, however, your doctor says you're overweight, you should calculate your total caloric needs as 24 calories per kilogram. You can divide those calories so the breakfast meal remains small by eating more calories at lunch, dinner, and in the frequent small snacks you have between breakfast and lunch, between lunch and dinner, and between dinner and bedtime.

An evening snack can be composed of a few crackers to make it equal to a half slice of bread and some protein put on the crackers. Peanut butter is actually the choice of many of my patients at the point before they go to bed. Yogurts are also available to you, but please be careful. Do not choose the yogurts that have the jellies or simple sugars in them. You're welcome to have all the plain yogurt you want, as long as you don't go over the total number of calories that you are allowed to eat.

What if you wake up hungry in the middle of the night? In that case, it would be fine to have a glass of milk, because it will prevent you from starving, going too long without eating, and therefore arriving at your next meal so hungry that you can't control yourself and may end up gobbling up too many carbohydrates. Frequent small feedings will help you stay on your diet.

You must measure your blood sugar when you wake up in the morning and one hour after beginning breakfast, lunch, and dinner. Chart these blood sugars on your record-keeping pages that your health-care team gave you, and chart all the foods that you eat. Please feel free to call your health-care team if you see that during the week when you're working on your own, your blood sugar is going outside the target range fasting of 90 and one hour after eating of 120. It isn't fair to the baby for you to go a long time with high blood sugars.

If your blood sugars stay within the target range, come back to your health-care team about a week later and show off your wonderful handiwork. Many times I look at a diary and see that a woman's blood sugars are actually beautifully low, never going above 100 or 110, and therefore she has the ability to tolerate more carbohydrate. At first, don't eat any of the extra carbohydrates you're allowed at breakfast. It's always a concern that that may be the hardest meal to handle. But at lunch and dinner perhaps another bread exchange might be tolerated so you could have a whole sandwich rather than just half a one. Indeed, if the blood sugar stays less than 120, your baby doesn't know or care what Mother puts into her mouth.

The way I usually experiment with giving back a

sweet fruit when my patients are dying for a banana or an orange is to use the afternoon as the experimental time. Eat the banana, then half an hour later measure your blood sugar. If your blood sugar is less than 120, then a banana can be used as an afternoon snack, likewise an orange. The reason I ask you to measure your blood sugar only half an hour after eating this single fruit is because without protein and fat, the sugars get into the bloodstream very quickly. In a mixed meal such as lunch or dinner the carbohydrates are slowed down by the fat content of the meal plan, and therefore the highest blood sugar is one hour after the meal. We want to see the highest blood sugars because that's the way we know exactly what the baby is experiencing. We don't want to look at just the best blood sugars. Those can't tell us whether the baby is getting sick and overweight.

Now I'm going to give you an opportunity to burn the sugars that you've eaten with a mild exercise program. Research has shown that exercise is a wonderful way to burn the sugar once you've consumed it. Of course, the human species could not have survived if exercise had been forbidden for a pregnant woman. How could the Neanderthal woman have run away from danger and perpetuate humankind if she had not been allowed to exercise during pregnancy or kept aborting every time she got up to do something? After all, in the olden days survival was dependent on moving and migrating. It makes sense that exercise has been a normal, healthy mode for pregnant women throughout the ages.

However, recent literature has shown that strenuous weight-bearing exercise may be difficult for a pregnant woman. When a woman tries to perform strenuous weight-bearing exercise such as running, energetic jogging, or stair climbing, what happens is the muscles around her uterus are exercised and irritate the womb so that it starts to contract. So premature labor may be a risk factor if a woman does weight-bearing exercise. This can also happen if she tries to bicycle, because the muscles around the uterus or womb are irritated; and even though she's not putting a lot of weight on her feet, the irritation is sufficient for the uterus to start contracting. With all the blood now existing in the legs, if the last little drop of blood is also cut off by the contraction or by the constricting of the blood vessels when the contraction occurs, the baby suffers and shows distress by slowing its pulse rate. So the best advice is not to burn the sugar by doing weight-bearing exercises or biking. If you do choose to do these exercises, it is a good idea to put your hand on your womb and feel whether it is tight or soft. (You want it to feel soft.) If it feels hard, that would be difficult for the baby, because once again, it means the baby is not getting a good blood supply. So, in general, you have permission to do whatever kind of exercise you want to do as long as your uterus stays soft.

Many women prefer to swim. Theoretically swimming should be an excellent form of exercise, for there is no weight bearing whatever with swimming and the muscles used are far away from the uterus and so the uterus would not be irritated. But to date we have not been able to test the baby or the uterus electronically because there are no waterproof devices for this experiment at the moment. So if you do want to swim, just make sure you test your own uterus with your hand to see that it is nice and soft, and then you can use swimming as your main way of exercise. However, if you don't have a pool in your backyard or access to a public pool, the best form of exercise for you is upper-arm exercise. Women who have very weak arms can work up a sweat just by lifting a couple of pounds in each arm. What I suggest you do is find a sturdy chair in your

house with a good back support and put it in front of
your TV set. Then start exercising at about five o'clock
in the evening when the news comes on. News programs
are usually half an hour long and the sports typically
come on twenty minutes into the news broadcast.
Therefore, if you exercise up to the sports report, you've
had a twenty-minute workout. American sports medicine
experts claim that twenty minutes of a cardiovascular
workout (which means that you are short of breath and
your pulse is racing) are sufficient exercise to burn sugar
and exercise the heart. So you only have to exercise from
the start of the news until the time the sports begin.

For your upper-arm exercise equipment, go to your
pantry and pull out two pounds of flour and two pounds
of sugar. (The containers should be about two pounds
each.) Sit firmly in your chair, hold a two-pound container in each hand, and, as you watch the news, lift first
the right arm, then the left arm. Lift the bag of flour or
sugar above your head and stretch way up to the ceiling.
Bring it back down to the level of your shoulder and
stretch the other arm, again pushing the bag of flour or
sugar way up to the ceiling. Alternate each arm about
five times and then push up both. It should be in a
rhythm as follows: Right only—1 and 2 and 3 and 4 and
5. Left only—1 and 2 and 3 and 4 and 5. And both—1
and 2 and 3 and 4 and 5. Goodness, I got short of breath
just saying that, fantasizing about lifting two pounds
with each arm!

I'd like you to sing "Row, row, row your boat" when
the sports come on, because if you can't finish the line
"Row, row, row your boat gently down the stream" in
one breath, then that's excellent because it means you're
short of breath and you're getting a good cardiovascular
workout. If you can complete the whole sentence or the
whole phrase without taking a breath, it means you don't

have enough weights on each arm and are not exercising sufficiently to burn sugar. So you should move up to five pounds for each arm.

On the other hand, if you can't get farther than five minutes into the news because you feel you're dying, stop and relax Go to your pantry the next day (don't try to force yourself on the same day), take out one-pound sacks of sugar or flour, or one-pound cans of tomatoes, and try this lower weight. If it becomes impossible to lift anything, perhaps you should start with no weights and just do hand raising, letting the weight of your hands be sufficient to start you off on this exercise program. Little by little you'll find yourself increasing the weights in order to complete the cardiovascular workout. After twelve sessions, you'll be absolutely amazed at how strong you are!

The other side effect of this exercise program is wonderful. You'll find that your one-hour-after-dinner blood sugar is miraculously low and you are, in fact, able to eat more and more carbohydrates. It's almost as though you don't have diabetes during dinner. If this is the case, maybe you'd like to exercise every day before dinner. It's sufficient, however, to exercise only three times a week to get an overall lowering effect.

The other thing you may want to do, if you're having trouble with your wake-up blood sugars, is to try exercising just before bed. You may find that this lowers the next morning's fasting blood sugar and helps you stay in the target range.

Using exercise as a treatment, therefore, can make your life not only easier, it may prevent you from needing insulin if you are borderline, tickling the upper limits of normal, and your health-care team is starting to suggest that perhaps you need an insulin injection.

If you've tried to stick to the diet and follow an exercise program but blood sugars still remain high, for the sake of your baby we have to move on to the next step. We can't use the pills that I prescribe for the elderly Type II or non–insulin-dependent diabetics because the pills cross the placenta and cause problems in the baby. The medicine gets in the baby's bloodstream, and the baby therefore can develop a very low blood sugar. So these pills really are counterindicated. Insulin given by injection does not cross the placenta. It can gently lower your blood sugars, and the baby doesn't know that you're taking insulin in order to make your blood sugars normal.

Unfortunately, we don't have any insulin you can drink; insulin will decompose in the stomach and will not get absorbed at all. Therefore, we must inject it. The truth of the matter is that an insulin injection is actually less painful than sticking your finger, and you're already sticking your finger four times a day. You'll be amazed that the needle on an insulin syringe hardly hurts at all. This will be your relieved response after your health-care team has taught you how to inject yourself correctly. The injection procedure is very simple, but you deserve to have an expert teach it to you so that your technique will be as perfect as possible. Poor technique can cause not only minor infection but also bruising, which increases the pain. A nurse educator will probably be the one to teach you how to inject. She'll show you places to insert the needle so that it's easy to get the insulin in under the skin. She'll teach you how proper technique is to clean the skin and to pinch up an inch of fat so that you actually can't feel the needle go in. This is called a counterirritant. You're pinching so hard that the pinch hurts more than the needle. You push in the insulin, and it's all finished.

The right dose of insulin is that dose that keeps your

blood sugars normal, so we usually suggest that we look at your blood sugar diary. Let's say you're having a terrible time with lunch, that no matter what you eat for your midday meal your blood sugar goes up, but all your other blood sugars are quite normal. Then your health-care team may prescribe an injection of a fast-acting insulin (called Regular) before lunch so you can eat a proper meal and yet still have normal blood sugars. The same could be true with your breakfast or your dinner. This process is called individualizing your insulin injection dosing. However, if you're having trouble with your wake-up blood sugar, if it's above 90 mg/dl on your own glucose monitor, then the best way to lower that number, if exercise before bed has not done the trick, is to take a dose of insulin called NPH. NPH is an intermediate eight-hour insulin, which is injected before bed as late as possible, because you only have eight hours until you have to have this insulin double-checked by a blood sugar. Eleven o'clock at night would mean you could sleep until seven o'clock the next morning. The dose of NPH is calculated based on your body weight and your week of gestation. Insulin usually is calculated to be 0.15 units per kilogram of body weight. If you weigh 60 kilos you multiply that times 0.15, which is nine units of insulin, and that would be your dose of NPH before bed.

Now when you try the insulin on for size, of course, you do test your blood sugar more often. If you need insulin for each meal, that is three injections a day, and insulin before bed makes four. You'll need to double-check the peaks of the insulin and the peaks of the food. So starting insulin usually means that the number of blood-sugar checks goes up to six a day—before each meal and one hour afterward. Then if the overnight blood sugars are not perfect, you'll need to do a blood sugar at bedtime and another in the middle of the night just to make sure that everything is going smoothly all night long.

There is one situation in which the daytime blood sugars are super but the overnight blood sugars still remain very, very high. In that particular case, your physician will probably push the insulin as hard as possible before bed to conquer your next-morning-fasting blood sugar. We never put into one injection more than forty units of insulin, because the insulin will decompose rather than get in the bloodstream if it is put in too large a puddle. So you may need two injections of NPH before bed if you're a very large woman, or you may need a 3 A.M. injection of Regular insulin as a sort of tack-on to try to get the next day's blood sugar normal. We see this problem in women who are more than 130 percent above ideal body weight when they are diagnosed with gestational diabetes. If you're in this special category, you need extra tender loving care by your health-care team because your insulin protocol will be a little more complicated. But it doesn't mean that your blood sugars can't be normal. It does mean that your baby will be absolutely normal because you are taking such good care of yourself.

When your baby is developing, your insulin requirements will increase as a result of the increased anti-insulin hormones coming from your placenta. As your baby grows, so your placenta grows and secretes more of these hormones. The normal response is to have the insulin requirement go up and up and up until it's time to have the baby. Then, about one week to ten days before you go into labor, you may find that your overnight insulin requirement actually starts dropping. This is because the uterus is practicing contractions and the contractions are like exercise. These contractions burn more sugar, so your overnight insulin requirement tends to drop as you get closer to going into labor.

Once labor begins, you'll need no more insulin. The exercise of labor completely uses up all your sugar. During labor you're not allowed to eat anything, so you won't have to worry about injections; and once the baby is born, 80 to 90 percent of the time your diabetes will go away. As soon as you feel the first contractions, throw away your insulin syringes and go to the hospital and have a healthy child. Your physician will help you measure your blood sugars in the hospital just to make sure you're getting the right intravenous solutions. One of the tricks may be for you to bring your own sugar-testing machine because we can't guarantee that the ones in the hospital are working perfectly all the time. Since you know your machine because you've been living with it, bring it along with enough sticks to keep you going for about twelve hours of labor. Measuring your blood sugar about every hour will assure that your baby will be absolutely normal. Normal blood sugars during labor and delivery vary between 60 and 120. This gives you plenty of room to swing, knowing that your blood sugars are normal and there is no problem with the baby. You probably won't need any insulin during the entire time of labor and delivery. Once your baby is born, he or she will be supernormal; therefore you'll be given the opportunity immediately to hold your baby and keep your baby with you.

We do recommend breast-feeding. Breast-feeding is a wonderful way to begin life. Ask your health-care team for proper nursing instructions. And don't worry; diabetes does not mean that you can't be a normal, healthy woman. You can breast-feed, even with diabetes. You just have to make sure that your blood sugars are normal. If you're one of the unlucky rare few who maintain high blood sugars after the baby is born, you'll need treatment at that time if you want to breast-feed. You don't want your blood sugars above 120 because the milk becomes too sweet. Sweet milk is also a way to provide extra calories to your baby, and you don't want your beautifully normal baby to get too fat from your sweet milk. If your blood sugars are above 120, your health-care team will advise you about the best methods to maintain your blood sugar in a normal range while you're breast-feeding.

About six weeks after the baby is born, or if you're breast-feeding when you first get your normal period, you will need a glucose-tolerance test. This will reassure you and document for your medical record that you do not have diabetes. One of the problems with a diagnosis of diabetes on your medical record is that the insurance provider sometimes increases its health-care costs. If you don't have diabetes, you need the proper way to confirm that you don't. That is done with a formal glucose-tolerance test. Your chart is then stamped as absolutely normal. However, if you don't lose weight and become fit between pregnancies, rest assured that during your subsequent pregnancies you have an 80 to 90 percent chance of having gestational diabetes again. As soon as you become pregnant the next time, you should bring your machine out of the closet, go buy some fresh reagent sugar sticks, and start measuring your blood sugar as you follow your normal meal plan. When you happen to have something extrasweet, measure your blood sugar again to see if it is below 120. If it is, you know you don't have diabetes yet. If, however, you ever see a blood sugar above 120, tell your health-care team you need the glucose-tolerance test, because gestational diabetes tends to come earlier in a pregnancy as we age and as we have more babies. So although you will be scheduled for the classic glucose test at about twenty to twenty-four weeks' gestation, or sometimes twenty-four to twenty-six weeks' gestation, right about in the middle of your pregnancy, if you see that your blood sugars are high at the beginning of the pregnancy, that would be a reason to call your health-care team and ask for help immediately.

One of the other suggestions I have for patients is: If you find your blood sugar goes above 120 if you eat something sweet, then I just automatically define you as having gestational diabetes and you don't have to bother doing the glucose tolerance test. After all, the reason for the test is just to get us started with diet and blood-sugar monitoring. If you're willing to do that based on your own testing and your own diagnostic skills, let's just go ahead and call you a gestational diabetic woman and begin the diet, the blood-sugar monitoring, the exercise program, and taking insulin if that is what you need to keep your blood sugars from going too high. You know what to do and how to do it. It seems unnecessary to take that drink to diagnose what you already know you have.

As we age, the prevalence of noninsulin-dependent diabetes increases. We already know that you have the genetic predisposition toward diabetes because you have had gestational diabetes. When you get older, there is a 60 percent chance you will develop Type II diabetes. There is, however, something you can do to change your fate. If after your pregnancies you become lean and fit, your chances of developing Type II diabetes in the future drop to less than 25 percent. So it's worth keeping up your skills of diet compliance and an exercise program after the babies are born. That way you may be able to keep the wolf of diabetes from your door. Developing diabetes is not just a nuisance but also is associated with other complications such as heart attacks, strokes, blindness, losing feet. I'm sure you're aware of all these complications because, intelligent woman that you are, you ran to the library to learn about gestational diabetes. At that time you undoubtedly read a whole chapter or maybe even a whole book about diabetes in general, so you know what happens to people with diabetes as they age if they don't take good care of themselves. With proper care, proper nutrition, and attention to keeping the blood sugar normal, none of these complications have to happen to you—after all, you want to be a great great-grandmother to the precious children you're bearing. So as you see, the diagnosis of gestational diabetes is actually a blessing. You've been blessed with new knowledge about diet, exercise, and metabolism, and you have a window on the future and can change your fate.

Congratulations and welcome to the club!

# Appendices

# $\mathscr{A}$ppendix A

## Recommended Reading

### Basic Books on Diabetes

Anderson, James, M.D. *Diabetes: A Practical New Guide to Healthy Living*, New York: Warner Books, 1981. This book explains Dr. Anderson's High Carbohydrate-Fiber Nutrition plan (HCF), which he began developing in 1974. His diet is particularly helpful for overweight Type II's, as it features very low-fat meals. It lowers blood glucose, weight, and cholesterol. Dr. Anderson was one of the original oat bran enthusiasts and contributed much research for lowering cholesterol with fiber.

Beaser, Richard, M.D., with Joan V. C. Hill, R.D., C.D.E. *The Joslin Guide to Diabetes.* New York: Simon & Schuster, 1995. This is the successor to the 12th edition (1989) of the classic *Joslin Diabetes Manual.* The Joslin Clinic in Boston, opened in 1898, is the oldest diabetes treatment center in the United States. The *Guide* is a "program for managing your treatment." It is truly up-to-the-minute for both Type I and Type II diabetes. It covers what and when to eat, how to monitor your blood sugars, how to administer insulin and oral medications, how to treat high and low blood sugar, how and when to exercise, and numerous day-to-day concerns of people with diabetes, as well as special occasions and events in your life.

Beaser, Richard S., M.D. *Outsmarting Diabetes.* Minneapolis: Chronimed, 1994. This book is based on the results of the ten-year Diabetes Control and Complications Trial (DCCT), which proved that tight control, as opposed to standard methods, greatly reduces the effects of diabetes and the risk of long-term complications.

It covers how to design such a program and adjust it to your lifestyle, how to avoid weight gain, how to use multiple daily injections or a pump, meal planning, exercise and psychological concerns. It gives specific instructions and describes a broad choice of programs. Every Type I can benefit from reading it.

Biermann, June, and Barbara Toohey. *The Diabetic's Book; All Your Questions Answered.* 3d edition. Los Angeles: Tarcher, 1994. The classic first book to read when you're diagnosed diabetic. As one young man wrote us, "Although you did not pull any punches, you did present the facts in a clear, sensible, and balanced manner. Your book has started me on a positive beginning." It's also a complete update for long-term and "born-again diabetics."

This new 1994 edition is totally updated with lots of brand-new material plus a special supplement on weight loss. As editor Daniel Malvin says, "There's a scoop on every page!"

———. *The Diabetic's Total Health Book.* 3d edition. Los Angeles: Tarcher, 1992. The book that proves you can have a chronic disease and yet be the picture of health, leading a vital, productive, and happy life. It shows you how to do this by focusing on your health rather than on your disease. Teaches you how to achieve a strong body, a tranquil mind, and a blithe spirit. There are entertaining and effective sections on reducing stress and raising your spirits with travel, laughter, and hugs. The new edition is thoroughly up-to-date to reflect the latest changes in diabetes therapy and features thirty-five of June and Barbara's personal favorite recipes.

———. *The Peripatetic Diabetic.* Revised edition. Los Angeles: Tarcher, 1984. Originally published in 1969, this is June and Barbara's first and most personal diabetes book, the one that tells how to overcome that initial fear and despair and move on to a more joyful, exciting, and healthy life than ever before. This edition was updated to bring you into the contemporary world of diabetes therapy. But the original book with all its crises and confusions is still there, exactly as it was written—and lived.

Curtis, Judy. *Living with Diabetic Complications.* Shippensburg, Pa.: Companion Press, 1993. This is a book about, for, and by people who are living with serious diabetic complications. It is full of sound, workable strategies for coping physically and emotionally and is very thorough on medical treatment options and sources of additional specialized help. The author has had Type I diabetes for forty-two years and has experienced vision impairment, kidney disease, heart disease, neuropathy, and an amputation. As part of her research, she sent out a questionnaire to hundreds of people with complications. Their responses and ideas connect this book with the reality of every kind of complications problem.

Etzwiler, Donnell D., M.D., ed., and others. *Learning to Live Well with Diabetes.* Revised edition. Minneapolis: International Diabetes Center, 1991. This is a very readable, easy-to-use, comprehensive manual on managing diabetes written by over twenty-five prominent experts. It reflects the latest medical advances, technologies, and research. There are over thirty chapters covering all aspects of self-care.

Fredrickson, Linda, M.A., R.N., C.D.E., ed. *The Insulin Pump Therapy Book; Insights from Experts.* Slymar, Calif.: MiniMed Technologies, 1995. A phenomenal book with the most timely and sophisticated information, not only for people using a pump for continuous insulin delivery but also for those who inject insulin. You can't learn too much about insulin if you are a user. Here eighteen leading diabetes experts, many with worldwide reputations, tell you what they know about setting insulin dosages, preventing hypoglycemia, exercise, insulin adjustment, carbohydrate counting, and even pregnancy. A true meet-the-experts book with answers galore to all the most confusing of problems.

Guthrie, Diana, R.N., C.D.E., Ph.D., and Richard A. Guthrie, M.D. *The Diabetes Sourcebook.* Revised edition. Los Angeles: Lowell House, 1995. This is a basic reference guide by a renowned husband and wife nurse and doctor team. Always in the forefront of diabetes therapy and education, they here present information on how to give yourself the best care. Very good on interacting with health professionals and family and friends.

Henry, Lester, Jr., M.D., with Kirk A. Johnson. *Black Health Library Guide to Diabetes.* New York: Henry Holt, 1993. The first guide written expressly for African Americans, one in every ten of whom has diabetes. Diabetes is the third leading cause of death in their racial group. This important book is by the Chief of Endocrinology at Howard University, a man with more than fifty years' experience treating and researching diabetes. His message to his people is, "If you respect diabetes, you can survive it." And his book tells them what they need to know to respect and survive it.

A sound, realistic, and up-to-date book, very clearly written and with a wonderful philosophy. A distinctive feature is the list of large drug companies who have programs to help low-income patients obtain medicine free of charge (including insulin). All must be contacted by your doctor, not by you.

Lodewick, Peter A., M.D. *A Diabetic Doctor Looks at Diabetes: His and Yours.* Waltham, Mass.: R. M. I. Corporation, 1993.

This totally rewritten edition of Dr. Lodewick's basic self-care book is head and shoulders—and pancreas—above the usual beginner's manual. Because he's had diabetes for twenty-five years and had thousands of diabetic patients in his practice, his perspective is realistic and refreshing. First off, he recognizes that "no two cases are alike." (What a breakthrough in medical thinking!) The range of topics covered is broad: everything from the overuse of insulin to diet options (big choice here) to dental health to pregnancy and impotence. The section on drinking distilled water is alone worth the price of the book.

Lowe, Ernest, and Gary Arsham, M.D., Ph.D. *Diabetes: A Guide to Living Well.* 2d revised edition. Minneapolis: Chronimed Publishing, 1992. A management guide for Type I's, written by two authors who've had diabetes for more than thirty-five years, plus a special chapter for women by Kathy Feste, a diabetic for over thirty years. The only book that gives individualized guidance in the sense that you're offered three programs of self-care: intensive, moderate, or loose. This is an all-inclusive book of concrete advice.

Milchovich, Sue K., R.N., C.D.E., and Barbara Dunn-Long, R.D. *Diabetes Mellitus: A Practical Handbook.* 6th revised edition. Palo Alto, Calif.: Bull Publishing Company, 1995. This is an easy-to-use and thorough explanation of diabetes and how to control it. It is very complete on diet and food choices and includes the entire Exchange Lists and sample meals plans for different calorie levels. Large type. A good beginning book.

Peterson, Charles, M.D., and Lois Jovanovic-Peterson, M.D. *The Diabetes Self-Care Method.* Los Angeles: Lowell House, 1990. This book was written by two of the foremost endocrinologists of the U.S. before the DCCT study, but they had already foreseen the advantages of the intensive therapy approach. This is a best-selling, state-of-the-art manual which focuses on normalizing blood sugar through self-testing and insulin adjustment.

Walsh, John, P.A., and Ruth Roberts, M.S. *Pumping Insulin.* 2d revised edition. San Diego, Torrey Pines Press, 1994. Many people in the Diabetes Control and Complications Trial that proved the benefits of tight control used a pump instead of syringes for their insulin. Written by a ten-year veteran pump-user, this new second edition of the classic book gives you all the information you need for deciding whether or not to go onto a pump and all the tools you need for the successful use of one.

But you don't have to be on a pump or even considering one to get a lot out of this book. To quote Dr. Lois Jovanovic-Peterson, "It's actually a complete 'How to Fix my Diabetes' in one wonderful book."

## Type II Diabetes

Monk, Arlene, R.D., C.D.E., and others. *Managing Type II Diabetes.* Revised edition. Minneapolis: Chronimed, 1996. This book is one of the first and best to deal exclusively with Type II diabetes. The new updated revised 2d edition offers the latest medical advances and sound practical advice. Written by prominent health-care experts of the International Diabetes Center. Will give you a complete understanding of your problem and tell you the steps to take to handle it.

Valentine, Virginia, R.N., M.S., C.D.E., June Biermann, and Barbara Toohey. *Diabetes Type II and What to Do.* Los Angeles: Lowell House, 1993. This latest and most-up-to-date book on Type II is accurate, practical, and, above all, compassionate. Its ongoing message is "Type II Diabetes Is Not a Character Flaw." Virginia Valentine, herself Type II, clearly explains the difference between those who are overweight and have insulin resistance (Type II-R) and those who are of normal weight but are deficient in insulin (Type II-D). Entertaining and packed with information. Type II's will love it, and, more important, it will make them love and care for themselves.

## Emotional Health and Stress

Edelwich, Jerry, and Archie Brodsky. *Diabetes: Caring for Your Emotions.* New York: Addison-Wesley, 1986. This book explores the deepest feelings of diabetics. It is told in the words of the people who lived through them. Outstanding chapters on sexuality, conflicts with health professionals, and family dynamics. Type II diabetics, who often get short shrift, are given as much attention as Type I's.

Rubin, Richard R., Ph.D., June Biermann, and Barbara Toohey. *Psyching Out Diabetes: A Positive Approach to Your Negative Emotions.* Los Angeles: Lowell House, 1992. Diabetes control can be 90 percent in your head. This exciting, breakthrough book helps you straighten out your head and get rid of the fear, denial, depression, grief, frustration, embarrassment, and guilt that block good diabetes control and a good life. Shows how to improve your perspective and enables you to look at your diabetic challenges in a completely different way. Dr. Rubin is on the faculty of the Johns Hopkins Medical School and has a private practice in Baltimore. He has counseled diabetic patients for over twenty years and has a diabetic son and sister. Dr. Rubin speaks clearly, directly, and without any psychological mumbo jumbo.

## Parents and Children

Betschart, Jean, M.N. R.N., C.D.E., and Susan Thom, R.D., L.D., C.D.E. *In Control.* Minneapolis: Chronimed, 1995. The only (and much-needed!) self-help book especially for teens with diabetes. Just published! Talks teen language and tells true stories. Full of realistic problems and workable solutions.

Covers all concerns, including birth control and sex, dating, parties and alcohol, career choice, parents and siblings, and above all staying in control. Delightfully illustrated.

Both authors got diabetes as teens themselves and have both become outstanding diabetes educators. Amazingly, both have been president of the American Association of Diabetes Educators. What more can we say? Go for it. It's awesome!

Betschart, Jean, M.N., R.N., C.D.E. *It's Time to Learn About Diabetes.* Revised edition. Minneapolis: Chronimed Publishing, 1995. This workbook on diabetes for children ages eight to ten years is creatively and professionally written by a highly experienced Certified Diabetes Educator of the Children's Hospital of Pittsburgh. Will truly help any child (or parent!) learn good diabetes self-care. Wonderfully illustrated. Fill-in quizzes for each chapter. A uniquely important book for home and diabetes education class use. Invaluable for the newly diagnosed child.

Folkman, Jane, R.D., and Hugo Hollerorth, Ed. D. *A Guide for Women with Diabetes Who Are Pregnant or Plan to Be.* Revised edition. Boston: Joslin Diabetes Center, 1996. Produced at the Pregnancy Clinic of the renowned Joslin Diabetes Center, this clearly written labor of love includes everything learned at the nation's first diabetes clinic to care for the distinctive needs of pregnant women with diabetes. The most complete manual available on the subject.

Cinykin, Sheri Cooper. *Next Thing to Strangers.* New York: Lothrop, Lee & Shepard, 1991. The first novel with a sixteen-year old *boy* with diabetes as a leading character; and even the fourteen-year-old heroine has a weight problem. The two meet while visiting their grandparents near Phoenix for the Christmas holidays. Both are from single-parent homes and both have unhappy lives. This is the engrossing story of how, facing problems together, Jody and Cass are strengthened by their experiences and emerge as winners. Speaks to teens in their own language. Engrossing!

Heegard, Marge, M.A., and Chris Ternand, M.D. *When a Family Gets Diabetes.* Minneapolis: DCI Publishing, 1990. This book uses art therapy to help children with diabetes and their families understand and express their feelings about the disease. The child and family members draw pictures that relate to certain aspects of diabetes and then discuss why they drew what they did. An excellent communication tool.

Johnson, Robert Wood, IV, Sale Johnson, Casey Johnson, and Susan Kleinman. *Managing Your Child's Diabetes.* New York: MasterMedia Limited, 1992. This book, written by a father, mother, and diabetic daughter, is a boon for parents of newly diagnosed children. The first chapter, by Casey Johnson, who was diagnosed at age eight, was written when she was twelve and is a little masterpiece of advice to all parents. The rest of the book is detailed information on blood-sugar control as well as how to deal with doctors and hospitals, teachers and schools, and the rest of the diabetic child's family. The last chapter, by Kenneth Farber, executive director of the Juvenile Diabetes Foundation International, is an encouraging look into the future.

Jovanovic-Peterson, Lois, M.D., with Morton B. Stone. *Managing Your Gestational Diabetes.* Minneapolis: Chronimed Publishing, 1994. Dr. Jovanovic-Peterson is one of the country's leading authorities on gestational diabetes (a temporary form of diabetes that appears during pregnancy). This book guides you through the steps to control your diabetes and reduce risks to yourself and your baby. Essential reading for mothers-to-be who develop this form of diabetes.

Loring, Gloria. *Parenting a Diabetic Child.* Los Angeles: Lowell House, 1993. This TV star and celebrity chairman of the Juvenile Diabetes Foundation has parented her diabetic son for over twelve years. This is a complex job, requiring expert technical information, psychological insight, and emotional support. Gloria provides all three for parents of diabetic children, leading you gently and authoritatively as only a mother who's been there can.

Martin, Ann M. *The Truth about Stacey.* New York: Scholastic, 1986. Number 3 of a popular series of books for eight- to twelve-year-old girls called the Baby-Sitters' Club. It is about seven girls who run a baby-sitting service in their hometown. Stacey has diabetes, and this story is about how she handles her disease. Very positive with accurate and nonintrusive diabetes information.

————. *Stacey's Emergency.* New York: Scholastic, 1991. The Baby-Sitters Club book number 43 in which Stacey gets overburdened with work and ends up in the hospital.

Meirelles, Janet, R.N., C.D.E., *Diabetes Is Not a Piece of Cake.* Lake Oswego, Oreg.: Lincoln Publishing, 1994. Finally, a book full of information and understanding for the long-ignored nondiabetic who shares life with a person with diabetes. Will open the lines of communication, smooth out conflicts, and thereby improve the relationship and ease the burden on both sides. Clearly written, up-to-date, detailed. Based on 300 questionnaires and Janet's professional experience. Valuable reference section full of timely where-to-find-it and how-to-handle it information.

Nemanic, Allison, R.N., B.A., and others. *Diabetes Care Made Easy.* Minneapolis: International Diabetes Center, 1992. This is a step-by-step guide for controlling diabetes. It is written for both children (six- to nine-year-olds) and adults and is *extremely* easy to read with many illustrations that make for clear understanding. Covers all the basics: taking insulin, what to eat, exercises, testing blood sugar, coping with emotions.

Roberts, Willo Davis. *Sugar Isn't Everything*. New York: Macmillan, 1987. The subtitle of this novel is *A Support Book, in Fiction Form, for the Young Diabetic*. A professional children's book writer who herself became diabetic as an adult, Willo Roberts turned her own new knowledge and experience into a factually sound, therapeutically up-to-date novel with an eleven-year-old girl as its heroine. Amy develops diabetes, struggles with it, learns how to handle it, and eventually accepts it. Engrossing and true to life. Every young diabetic can relate to this novel, and learn more and feel better for having read it. Good for parents, too.

## Cookbooks, Nutrition, Weight Loss, and Exchanges

Cooper, Nancy, R.D. *The Joy of Snacks*. Minneapolis: Chronimed, 1991. For Type II's, snacking six to ten times a day is actually better than eating three square meals. Type I's need handy snacks to prevent or treat low-blood-sugar episodes. Here's a book, written by an acclaimed dietitian, to help both types. Lots of muffin and cookie recipes and a large selection of popcorn treats and special snacks for kids. Two hundred delicious recipes with exchanges.

Finsand, Mary Jane. *The Complete Diabetic Cookbook*. New York: Sterling, 1987. Everything from snacks to sophisticated gourmet dishes packed into one slim volume. Includes ADA exchanges. Real food that is simple to prepare.

———. *Diabetic Cakes, Pies, & Other Scrumptious Desserts*. New York: Sterling, 1988. Another treasury of 200 formerly forbidden delights for people with diabetes and weight watchers. Even includes a Grand Marnier soufflé! Gives exchanges and calorie and carbohydrate counts.

———. *The Diabetic Candy, Cookie, and Dessert Cookbook*. New York: Sterling, 1982. Chemist-nutritionist Finsand gives you over two hundred recipes using sugar replacements. A treasure of thrills for dessertees. Even tells you how to make ice-cream cones. Contains twelve pie recipes, seventeen cake recipes, and forty-four cookie recipes.

————. *The Diabetic Chocolate Cookbook*. New York: Sterling, 1984. The luxury of chocolate in candies, cookies, cakes, pies, and puddings is here made possible for diabetics. Exchanges and calories are provided for each recipe.

————. *Diabetic Microwave Cookbook*. New York: Sterling, 1989. Almost three hundred recipes covering an amazing array of dining choices, with emphasis on protein dishes, all prepared quickly, easily, and healthily in a microwave.

————. *Quick and Delicious Diabetic Desserts*. New York: Sterling, 1992. Scores of recipes for pies and puddings, cakes and cookies, ice creams and tortes. Luscious treats that will augment any meal.

Franz, Marion, M.S., R.D. *Exchanges for All Occasions*. Minneapolis: Chronimed, 1993. Packed full of sound, authoritative guidance for diabetic eating. This new edition has the latest nutrition facts and recommendations, even the new Food Guide Pyramid and labeling system. Lists hundreds of foods not on the ADA exchange lists. Covers every eating situation (camping, children's parties, holidays) and most cuisines (Jewish, southwestern, vegetarian, etc.).

————. *Fast Food Facts*. 4th revised edition. Minneapolis: Chronimed, 1994. A newly revised and expanded pocket-size guide (four by six inches) for making the right food choices at fast-food restaurants. Gives complete nutritional information on over 1,500 menu offerings from the fifteen largest fast food chains. Has symbols to designate items high in salt, fat, or sugar.

Gilliard, Judy, and Joy Kirkpatrick, R.D. *Beyond Alfalfa Sprouts & Cheese*. Minneapolis: Chronimed, 1993. A healthy cookbook for all people with diabetes—vegetarian or not. Over 125 easy-to-prepare recipes using ingredients found in most grocery stores. Low in fat and calories; not heavy in oils, nuts, seeds, cheese, and egg yolks like many vegetarian dishes. Emphasis is on fresh, high-quality ingredients and, most of all GOOD TASTE! Includes exchanges.

Gilliard, Judy, and J. Kirkpatrick. *Guiltless Gourmet.* Wayzata, Minn.: Diabetes Center, Inc., 1987. By a dietitian and a diabetic trained in classic French cuisine. This book has sophisticated recipes from all over the world, all computer analyzed for the diabetic diet. All are low in fat, cholesterol, sugar, and calories.

Hess, Mary Abbott, R.D., F.A.D.A., M.S., assisted by Jane Grant Tougas. *The Art of Cooking for the Diabetic.* 3d ed. Chicago: Contemporary Books, 1996. This could be called the diabetic person's *Joy of Cooking* because it has everything you need to know to understand the diet, plan and prepare delicious meals and snacks, and love doing it! Nondiabetics who share the meals won't believe they're on the diabetic diet. Contains 375 recipes that are low in saturated fats and sugar.

Juliano, Joseph, M.D., and Dianne Young. *The Diabetic's Innovative Cookbook.* New York: Henry Holt, 1994. Dr. Juliano, who's had diabetes for over thirty years and been blind for nine years, collaborates with a professional chef in a book of positive philosophy and zesty food that is low in fat and heart-healthy. One hundred and forty-five recipes in all plus Dr. Juliano's personal, practical advice on such vital subjects as parties, holiday food, desserts, sweeteners, fiber, and the role of family and friends.

Kruppa, Carole. *Free and Equal Cookbook.* 2d edition. Chicago: Surrey Books, 1994. The original, highly popular cookbook featuring all recipes with Equal (NutraSweet). The author grew up in a French family and does not sacrifice good taste in these 150 low-calorie and sugar-free recipes. Includes break-fast treats, appetizers, soups, salads, entrees, desserts, beverages, and jams. Gives calorie counts and exchanges for all recipes.

————. *Free and Equal Dessert Cookbook*. Chicago: Surrey Books, 1992. One hundred and fifty quick and delicious low-calorie desserts and sweet treats all using the sweetener Equal (NutraSweet). All recipes are also low-salt and low-cholesterol. Includes exchanges and calories.

LeShane, Patricia. *Vegetarian Cooking for People with Diabetes*. Revised and expanded edition. Summertown, Tenn.: Book Publishing Company, 1994. Over 100 true vegan recipes without dairy products or eggs, emphasizing low-fat cooking. Soy milk used for protein, instead of milk along with nuts, grains, and legumes (beans, lentils, garbanzos, soybeans, etc.). Sweeteners used are small amounts of blackstrap molasses or honey. No white flour or sugar. Sample dishes include: grainburgers, millet with tofu and mushrooms, soybean mushroom pilaf, nondairy scalloped potatoes, and pintos and pasta, apple-oat drop cookies, and rice pudding. The recipes are easy to prepare with Exchanges and fat percentages given for each.

Majors, Judith S. *Sugar Free Good and Easy; Sugar Free Goodies; Sugar Free Kids' Cookery*. Milwaukie, Ore.: Apple Press, 1987, 1987, 1989. Finally back in print, three books approved by the Oregon affiliate of the ADA and written by a diabetic woman who confesses she "lives to eat." All recipes are simple and quick. *Goodies* is for those with a sweet tooth—pies, cookies, jams, ice creams. *Good and Easy* has breads, salads, main dishes—everything for variety and good meals. *Kids' Cookery* has recipes with child appeal that are simple enough for young diabetics to prepare. Exchanges in each book.

Marks, Betty. *Microwave Diabetic Cookbook*. Chicago: Surrey Books, 1991. Over 130 fast, sugar-free recipes, all high in taste but low in fat, cholesterol, sodium, and calories. You can make a delicious meal in fifteen minutes or less thanks to the busy author, who is a literary agent, a prizewinning ballroom dancer, and an insulin-dependent person with diabetes.

Natow, Annette, Ph.D., R.D., and Jo Ann Heslin, R.D. *Diabetes Carbohydrate and Calorie Counter*. New York: Pocket, 1991. Gives carbohydrate, calorie, and fat count in grams for 3,000 foods from Abalone to Zucchini. Includes takeout and frozen items. Excellent guidelines for designing an eating plan for Type II diabetes.

———. *The Fat Counter*. New York: Pocket, 1993. Fat is the enemy of health; fat is the particular enemy of people with diabetes, especially Type II's. Among other things, it interferes with the action of insulin. This handy book gives the data needed to learn how to avoid it. Fat and calorie values given for over 10,000 foods, including packaged and frozen foods, thirty-six fast food chains, and prepared recipes and snacks. A bible of healthy avoidance.

Polin, Bonnie, and Frances Giedt. *The Joslin Diabetes Gourmet Cookbook*. New York: Bantam, 1993. Created under the aegis of the respected Joslin Clinic, this is a glorious collection of over 530 fabulous recipes appropriate for people with diabetes (low in fat, cholesterol, sugar, and salt) as well as those with cardiovascular problems and those who are healthy and want to stay that way.

Both authors have diabetes and a passion for good food. They use the best of healthy and sophisticated ingredients— radicchio, jicama, basmati rice, chanterelles, etc. Many ethnic dishes including Chinese, Mexican, Middle Eastern, North African. One hundred meal-planning and kitchen tips, many you can't find even in Julia Child, like how to seed a pomegranate.

Robertson, Laurel, Carol Flinders, and Brian Ruppenthal. *The New Laurel's Kitchen.* Berkeley: Ten Speed Press, 1986. *Laurel's Kitchen* has always been our favorite vegetarian cookbook. The new *Laurel* has the same inspiring philosophy and new recipes that open vistas of dining joy and health. Tells how to increase fiber and cut back on fat. Sections on cooking for children, elders, pregnant women, and athletes. Also now available in the abridged version: *Laurel's Kitchen Recipes.*

Ulene, Art, M.D. *The NutriBase Guide to Carbohydrates, Calories & Fats in Your Food.* Garden City, N.Y.: Avery Publishing Group, 1995. This is the most complete and handy listing of carbohydrates, calories, and fats in foods so far published—30,000 products in all. It includes whole foods, processed foods, and brand-name items. Very well cross-referenced and very clear about serving sizes. There are 682 pages of data in pocketbook size.

Warshaw, Hope, M.M.Sc., R.D. *Healthy Eater's Guide to Family & Chain Restaurants.* Minneapolis: Chronimed, 1993. The subtitle of this amazing new book is "What to Eat in Over 100 Restaurant Chains Across America." It gives you the best bets and shows how to put healthier and tasty meals together in ten different categories of chains: burger, chicken, dessert/ice cream, dinner houses, family and Mexican restaurants, pizza, sandwiches and subs, seafood, and steak houses. A groundbreaking book.

    In the Put It All Together sections there are sample meals with total exchanges. For all foods it gives calories, carbohydrates, protein, fat, cholesterol and sodium.

Warshaw, Hope S., M.M.Sc. *The Restaurant Companion.* Chicago: Surrey Books, 1990. The first book to focus entirely on restaurant dining. Shows how to make appropriate healthy choices for eight ethnic cuisines, including Mexican, Chinese, Italian, and Thai, as well as for American and fast-food restaurants. Also gives advice for salad bars, brunches, and airline meals. Describes ingredients in typical dishes and gives exchanges for recommended choices.

Waterhouse, Debra, M.P.H., R.D. *Outsmarting the Female Fat Cell.* New York: Hyperion, 1993. The first weight-control program specifically designed for women. Based on scientific data and the author's experiences in her private practice as a registered dietitian. Designed to get women's fat cells to burn, not store, fat. Shows how to stop starving and start eating by fat-proofing your diet. Includes this sound advice: Find your comfortable and healthy weight that is not determined by society but by your body type and genetics.

## Exercise

Bailey, Covert, and Lea Bishop. *The Fit or Fat Woman.* Boston: Houghton Mifflin, 1987. Exercise guru Bailey attacks the problem that women get fat more easily than men. Deals with the medical, dietary, and hormonal factors that drive fat up in women—and how to counteract them. Advice on strength building, aerobic exercise, and diet. Covers the social pressures women face and has special sections on depression, PMS, anorexia, and bulimia.

Bailey, Covert. *The New Fit or Fat.* Boston: Houghton Mifflin, 1991. The essential message of this well-researched breakthrough book is that overweight people should concentrate on losing body fat, not pounds. Bailey says that fat people often eat less than skinny people and the only way they can lose body fat is through exercise that changes their metabolism. Exercise resets all the body mechanisms to lower body fat. His message: "The ultimate cure for obesity is exercise." Other valuable books for following Bailey's program are *Fit or Fat Target Diet* and *Fit or Fat Target Recipes.*

Gordon, Neil F., M.D., Ph.D., M.P.H. *Diabetes: Your Complete Exercise Guide.* Champaign: Human Kinetics, 1993. Shows how a regular exercise program combined with proper nutrition and medication can help people with diabetes control their disease and improve their health. Describes the exercises and activities that are most beneficial for increasing flexibility, strength, and aerobic fitness as well as reducing the risk of complications.

Graham, Claudia, Ph.D., C.D.E., June Biermann, and Barbara Toohey. *The Diabetes Sports and Exercise Book.* Los Angeles: Lowell House, 1995. This modernization of the popular 1977 book, which was based on the sports experiences of 168 diabetic exercise enthusiasts, contains all the new scientific and technical information unavailable eighteen years ago. It's everything you need to know to gain the marvelous therapeutic effect of exercise along with all the fun it brings into your life. Tells how to use sports to best advantage and how to avoid any possible negative outcomes. Special chapters for children, those with complications, and the elderly. Will inspire and motivate you not to miss out on what has been called the "toy department of life."

# $\mathcal{A}$ppendix B

## Desirable Weight for Height Chart

Since this federal chart applies to both men and women, women should fall at the lower end of the weight range (they have less muscle and bone than men).

| Height* | Ages 19 to 34 | 35 and over |
|---------|---------------|-------------|
| 5'0" | 97–128 | 108–138 |
| 5'1" | 101–132 | 111–143 |
| 5'2" | 104–137 | 115–148 |
| 5'3" | 107–141 | 119–152 |
| 5'4" | 111–146 | 122–157 |
| 5'5" | 114–150 | 126–162 |
| 5'6" | 118–155 | 130–167 |
| 5'7" | 121–160 | 134–172 |
| 5'8" | 125–164 | 138–178 |
| 5'9" | 129–169 | 142–183 |
| 5'10" | 132–174 | 146–188 |
| 5'11" | 136–179 | 151–194 |
| 6'0" | 140–184 | 155–199 |

*Height without shoes; weight without clothes.*

Adapted from the U.S. Department of Agriculture and the U.S. Department of Health and Human Services' publication *Nutrition and Your Health: Dietary Guidelines for Americans.* 3d ed. Washington, D.C.: U.S. Government Printing Office, 1990.

# $\mathcal{I}$ndex

275

# $\mathcal{A}$bout the Authors

DR. LOIS JOVANOVIC-PETERSON is a senior scientist at The Sansum Medical Research Foundation in Santa Barbara and is a Clinical Professor of Medicine in the Division of Endocrinology at the University of Southern California in Los Angeles. Dr. Jovanovic-Peterson has written hundreds of articles and textbooks in the field of diabetes and pregnancy. In 1995, she received the Outstanding Physician Clinician Award from the American Diabetes Association. She was the chair of the Diabetes and Pregnancy Council of the American Diabetes Association, 1989–1991, and currently is the president of the California Affiliate of the American Diabetes Association. Dr. Jovanovic-Peterson's work in the field of diabetes and pregnancy has become the mainstay of therapy for all diabetic pregnant women. Because of her research, diabetic women now have the same chances as nondiabetic women to have a healthy infant.

JUNE BIERMANN and BARBARA TOOHEY have written fifteen books and hundreds of magazine articles on diabetes in the many years of their collaboration. They began writing about diabetes in 1969, after June was diagnosed as diabetic in 1967. Since then, they have been speakers at diabetes programs and seminars, as well as at local and national meetings of the American Diabetes Association, and have made numerous appearances on TV and radio talk shows. June and Barbara were the founders of the

SugarFree Centers (now Diabetes Self Care), a national source of diabetic products. They are currently codirectors of Prana Publications in Van Nuys, California, publishers of *The Diabetic Reader*.